Springer Wien New York

Wolfgang Seeger

Endoscopic Anatomy of the Third Ventricle

Microsurgical and Endoscopic Approaches

In collaboration with
J. P. Warnke, St. Rosahl, and A. Weyerbrock

SpringerWienNewYork

Professor Dr. med. Wolfgang Seeger
Prof. em für Neurochirurgie der Universität Freiburg i. Br.
Au, Federal Republic of Germany

© 2006 Springer-Verlag/Wien
Printed in Austria

SpringerWienNewYork is a part of Springer Science+Business Media
springeronline.com

Data conversion, Figure reproduction, Printing and Binding:
Druckerei Theiss GmbH, St. Stefan, Austria, www.theiss.at

Printed on acid-free and chlorine-free bleached paper

SPIN: 11599586

With 47 Figures

Library of Congress Control Number: 2006920092

ISBN-10 3-211-31177-7 SpringerWienNewYork
ISBN-13 978-3-211-31177-6 SpringerWienNewYork

Preface

Endoscopical surgery of the third ventricle has been applied for many years by transcerebral routes, especially as ventriculo-cisternostomies by opening the floor of the third ventricle. These surgeries were carried out either free-hand, or using stereotaxy or – later on – neuronavigation. Spaceoccupying vascular and other lesions, such as tumors or cysts located in the third ventricle, were usually eliminated by microsurgical approaches. These approaches were carried out mainly by approaches along the extracerebral midline structures or close to them. Midline approaches, especially approaches along the falx crossing the Corpus callosum, are less invasive than transcerebral approaches. Extracerebral midline approaches are variable in extent and direction of the approach, transcerebral approaches are less variable. A further aspect is the sagittal extension of the third ventricle in the midline so that it can be reached easily by midline surgical approaches. A combination of microsurgery (for the extraventricular part of surgery) and endoscopy (for the intraventricular part of surgery) has been performed in the recent years. However, the appliance of this combined technique is not common for the following reasons:

– Rare indications for surgery of midline structures
– Technical aspects
  Using flexible endoscopes it is possible to inspect all segments of the third ventricle. But surgical manipulations are only possible in a straight direction. Flexible endoscopes are not available in all neurosurgical departments at this point of time.
– Anatomical aspects
– Anatomical details are well known for the microsurgical approaches. However, numerous common variants of the anatomy of the extraventricular routes are still unknown.

In this book anatomical aspects important for combinations of microsurgical and endoscopical approaches are presented and illustrated. Numerous common anatomical variants are demonstrated with reference to their impact for the surgical technique. Combinations of both surgical techniques are called "surgical" in this book, except for procedures, which are exclusively microsurgical or endoscopical procedures. These techniques are called "microsurgical", or "endoscopical", respectively.

The authors successor in Freiburg, Professor Dr. J. Zentner, made available rooms and materials for the anatomical dissections and demonstrations, as he has been doing for more than 7 years of his chairmanship in Freiburg. His vice-chairman Privatdozent Dr. S. Rosahl, has demonstrated endoscopical and microsurgical operations during cadaver head dissection.

The author found a good translator in Dr. A.Weyerbrock, who edited the manuscript and helped to improve numerous neurosurgical aspects of presentation of this book.

I am grateful to Mrs. E. Rotermund, Professor Zentner's secretary for typing and preparing the final edition of the manuscript.

I would especially like to thank the Springer-Verlag Wien New York for the continuous good cooperation, help and excellent production of this book.

Wolfgang Seeger

Contents

Overview (Fig. 1)

Using natural CSF-spaces close to the midline, there are 4 types of surgical approaches. Transcerebral approaches are not described here.

Anatomical Basis (Figs. 2 to 15)

Target areas, overview (Fig. 2)

The spatial imagination of the three-dimensional structures of the 3rd ventricle and its adjacent structures can be facilitated, if a cast of the ventricle (Fig. 2 A) is compared with the shapes of the adjacent structures of the 3rd ventricle (Fig. 2 B)

Details (Figs. 3 to 15)

Bulgings and excavations of the intraventricular relief may be used for landmarks. *Each bulging corresponds to a bulging of an adjacent structure:*
– Commissura ant. and post.
– Corpora mamillaria
– Columnae fornicis (partes liberae)
– Plexus chorioideus
– Adhesio interthalamica (inconstant)
There are two types of excavations:
– Excavations of thinwalled segments of the 3rd ventricle, that are Recessus suprapinealis, Sulcus prae- and Recessus postmamillaris
– Excavations which result from thickening of adjacent structures in the excavated segments of the wall of the 3rd ventricle: Recessus opticus, Recessus infundibuli, Recessus pinealis.

None of all cerebral ventricles present as many excavations as the 3rd ventricle. It is explained by the development of the optic and incretory system, using the wall of the excavations for the development of Retina, Nn. optici, Corpus pineale, and hypophyseal stalk. Sensory areas for the perception of light, for adapting the color of skin to the color of surroundings (Hyla arborea, e.g.), and the residuals of optic functions in Corpus pineale in many vertebrata, are well known by zoologists and anatomists.

Thin walls of excavations can be used for endoscopical approaches, especially after the widening of the wall of the ventricle. But here, the excavations are flattened, too. Now other landmarks may better to be used: Recessus opticus, Recessus infundibuli, Corpora mamillaria, Aquaeductus, the commissures, and Foramen interventriculare

Anterior segment of the third ventricle (Figs. 3 and 4)

The anterior area of the 3rd ventricle can be overseen well by a view from a posterior direction, the posterior area by a view from an anterior direction (according to the supracerebellar and to the translaminar approach, especially, if a flexible endoscope is not available).

The anterior area of the 3rd ventricle presents all details of Foramina interventricularia: Columnae fornicis (Partes liberae) are plexus-free and build up the reliefs of the anterior, medial and lateral segments of the foramina. **These important allocortical structures can be damaged especially by transforaminal surgical approaches.** The posterior wall relief of Foramen interventriculare is build up by Plexus chorioideus. Plexus chorioideus transits from Plexus of the lateral ventricle into Plexus of the 3rd ventricle. It encloses the transition of V. thalamostriata into V. cerebri interna, and its connection with V. septi pellucidi. Anterior from this point V. septi pellucidi penetrates Columna fornicis after its subependymal course in Septum pellucidum.

The transition of Columna fornicis into Corpus fornicis is defined by the posterior wall of Foramen interventriculare. Here the plexus-free Columna fornicis transits into the plexus-connected Corpus fornicis. The transition of Pars libera fornicis into Pars tecta is located immediately underlying the lateral margin of Foramen interventriculare. Here the penetration point of Columna fornicis is recognizable by looking into the foramen from a dorsal direction (according to the transforaminal approach, e.g.) or from a posterior direction (according to the supracerebellar approach, e.g.), as seen in Figs. 3A and 3B. Its continuation (Pars tecta, dotted lines), ends in Corpus mamillare.

Both Columnae fornicis are enclosing a trigonal-shaped area. Its base is built by Commissura ant. Its tip is located at the point of connection of Rostrum, Septum pellucidum and the fusion of both Columnae fornicis.

For anatomical base see Fig. 3A and B, for surgical aspects see text page 24 and Figs. 45B' and 47B).

The trigonal zone is a tabu zone for surgical manipulations: Danger for irreversible postoperative psychological deficits! Common variants of Columnae fornicis and of plexus of the 3rd ventricle are shown in Fig. 3:
– Asymmetry of Columnae fornicis (C')
– Duplication of Plexus chorioideus (D')

A summary of the anterior area of the 3rd ventricle and its surrounding structures is given in a simplified copy of an axial MRT-slice (Fig. 4): Falx is smaller than in dorsal Falx segments. The subarachnoid space between Falx and Lamina terminalis is long. In this slice of MRT the subarachnoid space is interrupted by the basal segment of Genu corporis callosi. Aa. cerebri antt. (A2) and its branches are seen anterior and posterior from the transectional shape of Genu corporis callosi. Most important intraventricular structures are the anterior-commissure-Fornix-complex, Chiasma-infundibular-mamillar-segment, and, for ventriculo-cisternostomy, the area between Recessus infundibuli and Corpora mamillaria (see topogram in Fig. 5).

Posterior segment of the 3rd ventricle (Figs. 5 and 19)

In Fig. 5 MRT is presented as in Fig. 4, with accentuation of the occipital area. The topographical relationships are more difficult to understand than it is in the frontal area.

At the MRT-slice, Splenium is transsected close to its inferior limit. The vein of Galen is transsected twice, because it is running around the inferior posterior surface of Splenium. This projection is helpful for spatial imagination:

Recessus suprapinealis basally from this is presented. It overlaps incompletely Corpus pineale. Inferior to Recessus suprapinealis the pineal recessus is recognizable. Commissura post. is bulging against the ventricular lumen, basally from Recessus pinealis. It overlaps the entrance of Aquaeductus.

Lesions of this area by surgery, e.g., may be followed by severe vegetative and psychological deficits.

Adjacent structures of the 3rd ventricle (Figs. 6 to 15)

1. Corpus callosum (Fig. 6)

The approximately length of Corpus callosum is measured 8 cm, but length and configuration are variable. A shortening may occur, if Genu, or the middle segment, or Splenium corporis callosi are thickened. This variability should be considered regarding MRT's, if the interventricular foramina are not exact defined. The foramina may be masked by a hyperplastic plexus or they may be compressed by pathological factors. In normal conditions, the distance measurements of Genu corporis callosi and Foramen interventriculare vary approximately between 4 and 6cm. If the preoperative defining of Foramen interventriculare is not precise, the usual defining by the distant measurement to Genu corporis callosi is correct as well. Here the relationship with Bregma and Corpora mamillaria is helpful, as given in the chapter of transforaminal surgical approaches (Fig. 22).

2. Addendum for 1 (Fig. 7)

Rostrum corporis callosi and Lamina terminalis (Fig. 7)
Rostrum corporis callosi is especially important regarding its topographical relationships with Allocortex:
– Area subcallosa
– Gyrus rectus, posterior segment
– Commissura anterior-Columnae-fornicis-complex

Severe psychological deficits may occur if these structures are damaged.

3. Fornices (Figs. 9 to 11)

There are 4 segments of Fornix:
– Columna fornicis
– Corpus fornicis
– Crus fornicis
– Fimbria fornicis
The only commissure of the fornix is Commissura fornicis. Septum pellucidum forms an anatomical and functional unit with Columna fornicis (Pars libera) and Corpus fornicis. Crura and Commissura fornicis are fused with the inferior surface of Corpus callosum.

Intraventricular surface of Fornices
– Columna fornicis
Pars tecta (between the area of For. interventriculare and Corpus mamillare) is located subependymally. This segment and Columna fornicis, Pars libera (surrounding Foramen interventriculare) are the only plexus-free segments of Fornix.

– Corpus fornicis
is called the beginning plexus-connected segment of Fornix. The plexus begins at the posterior wall of the interventricular foramen, coming from the plexus of the 3rd ventricle, and continuing into the lateral ventricle

Fornix is connected with plexus by Taenia fornicis. Plexus is connected at its medial basal part with Lamina affixa thalami and it continues to Velum interpositum by the richly vascularized Taenia chorioidea. A variable number of mostly thin veins, medial septal veins, are running from Septum pellucidum in a subependymal course to the dorsal surface of Fornix, then to Plexus chorioideus of the lateral ventricle, to Thalamus, to Tela chorioidea of the 3rd ventricle and they are entering the inner cerebral veins

– Crura fornicis
Posterior from the Fornices – Septum-pellucidum – complex, Fornices are dividing into Crura fornicis, whose course diverges from the midline into a lateral basal direction. It

builds the medial basal segment of Atrium ventriculi. Behind this segment it continuously reduces in diamater

– Fimbria fornicis
This small segment is the continuation of Fornix to Cornu inf.
Extracerebral surface of Fornices
The extracerebral surface of Fornices is the roof of Fissura transversa. Fissura transversa is interposed between Fornices and Velum interpositum. Fornices and Fissura transversa are nearly congruent. Both shapes are triangular, as well as Velum interpositum. The fornical compartiment is built by Crura fornicis with its divergent courses. Crura fornicis are fused with Corpus callosum, as well as Commissura fornicis, which connect them as a thin layer. This is a small area, normally. A median transection of Corpus callosum immediately anterior from Splenium will endanger Crura fornicis. Here an exact division between Crura fornicis by splitting of the small Commissura fornicis is problematic under normal circumstances. But it is not problematic at two common variants of Fornices: Prefixed Fornix and Fornices of Cavum Vergae (3.2.)

3.1. Fornix and Septum pellucidum (Fig. 9)

Columnae fornicis
Transversal cadaver brain dissections present a circular shaped tract of white matter. This tract is enclosed by a cap-like gray matter which is a thickened continuation of Septum pellucidum.
This area is a tabu zone for surgical resections.
Danger for psychological deficits!
Fornix and Septum pellucidum are one common functional and anatomical system. Tumors and other lesions which develop slowly, may destroy wide parts of both structures, even bilateral, without the development of psychological deficits. This is not to be expected after acute traumatic lesions, and after surgical manipulations.

Columnae and Corpora fornicis
are connected with Septum pellucidum, until it ends at a common fusion of Septum, Fornix, and Corpus callosum. Even the midline-guiding Cavum septi pellucidi ends here. Posterior from this point, both Fornices are dividing and running into a lateral basal direction. These segments are called Crura fornicis

3.2. Crura and Commissura fornicis (Figs. 9 to 11)

This area is triangular-shaped and fused with the inferior surface of Corpus callosum. The anterior tip of Commissura fornicis is located at the dividing point of Crura fornicis in the midline. Its posterior limit area is the transversal connection with the inferior anterior limit of Splenium corporis callosi. If the dividing point of Crura fornicis is located anterior from this typical area, it may be called prefixed Fornix (Fig. 9). If Fornices and Septum pellucidum are widened in a posterior dorsal and in a posterior basal direction, surrounded by a thin-walled Splenium (Cavum Vergae), then Cavum septi pellucidi is dilated or it is dilated at its posterior segment. Both variants, the prefixed Fornices as well as Cavum Vergae, present a widening of Commissura fornicis into a longitudinal and into a lateral direction. This is a favorable precondition for splitting Corpus callosum in the area of the midline without endangering the far lateral located Crura fornicis. Excepted is the anterior limit area of the commissura at prefixed Fornices. Immediately anterior from this area the cavum of Septum pellucidum often ends with a little dilation, not only at prefixed

Fornices (Fig. 9B and B', see a'). This is a favorable precondition for the inter-fornical approach.

4. Splenium and Tectum (Fig. 12)

Cisternae ambientes, Cisterna tecti, the cistern of the galenic vein, and Fissura trans-versa are compartments of only one common subarachnoidal space. All these cisterns contain a variable number of Trabeculae and vessels, especially veins, which may hinder surgical approaches.

5. Cisterna tecti and Fissura transversa (Figs. 13 and 14)

Multiple Trabeculae of Cisterna tecti require precise dissections. Vessels must be loosened and shifted aside. The tectal structures (Colliculi tecti, Corpus pineale, Nn. trochleares) are visible now. If necessary, the opening must be widened until the galenic cistern, Fissura transversa or Cisterna ambiens of one or each sides are visible. **Cave loosening of Corpus pineale!** Its connections with Thalamus (Habenula), with commissura posterior (contain-ing Commissura habenularum), and further structures close to the entrance of Aquaeduc-tus may be endangered. This is a tabu zone for surgical manipulations.

The entrance of Aquaeductus is not to be seen by an occipito-dorsal view direction. Us-ing a flexible endoscope, it can be visualized. At anatomical cadaver brain or cadaver head dissections, a probe can be introduced superior from the posterior commissure and close to it. If the probe appears inferior to Corpus pineale and superior from Tectum, then it has penetrated the thin wall between Corpus pineale and Commissura post. (con-taining Commissura habenularum).
Via falsa!

In a historical presentation (Fig. 13B) a damage of the wall of the 3rd ventricle between Corpus pineale and Commissura posterior is demonstrated. Microanatomical structures are seen in histological slices of fiber presentations (Zuleger and Staubesand 1977), Fig. 14 presents a sectional enlarged indian ink copy.

6. Vessels of Cisterna ambiens, Cisterna tecti, and Fissura transversa/Velum interpositum (Fig. 15)

– Arteries: Aa. chorioideae are originating from A. cerebri post. at the lateral segment of Cisterna ambiens. It are running in a dorso-medial direction after dividing in nu-merous fine branches. Dorsal from Habenula these branches are dividing in a medial and in a lateral bundle. The medial one is running along the galenic vein and along the inner cerebral veins. The lateral one diverges and is feeding Plexus chorioideus of the lateral ventricle and Thalamus, along Taenia chorioidea. Some fine branches of the main bundles are feeding Tectum (In the past: "Aa. quadrigeminae").
– Veins are located close to the midline. They are often divided in two or more branches. Superficial veins are Vv.cerebellares superficiales and V. (Vv.) supracul-minalis(es). Located in the depth are V.(Vv.) cerebellaris(es) praecentralis(es). It are originating from Cerebellum between Velum medullare ant. and Lobulus cerebel-laris praecentralis and/or between Lobulus cerebellaris praecentralis and its over-lapping lobuli.
Vv. tecti are running in a dorso-medial direction. All these veins are entering the galenic vein in the midline area, except V. basalis (Rosenthal). Rosenthal's vein is

originating from a convolute of veins between Uncus and the anterior area of Cornu inf.. Its feeders are different inferior ventricular veins, deep sylvian veins, the interpeduncular vein and lateral mesencephalic as well as basal thalamic veins. Rosenthal's vein is a singular vein or it is splitted in numerous fine and larger veins.

Rosenthal's vein is running close to the midbrain and Pulvinar, in contrast to A.cerebri post., which is running transcisternal. Rosenthal's vein enters the galenic vein or V. cerebri int.. Its main feeding branch, V. mesencephalica lat., is located at the posterior rim of Crus cerebri. It connects the Rosenthal-vein with V. petrosa sup. and may be connected with lateral pontine and cerebellar veins. This should be considered by surgery at the roof of the 3rd ventricle.

Surgical Approaches (Figs. 16 to 47)

Approaches transcrossing Lamina terminalis – translaminar approaches (Figs. 16 to 20)

Principles of surgical approaches (Fig. 16)

These approaches transcross the interhemispheric space in its frontopolar segment. The intradural part of these approaches begins in the area of a frontopolar bundle of bridging veins, which should be spared. These veins are draining the frontopolar and frontobasal cortex (Kaplan et al. 1976). Rostrally from it Sinus sagittalis sup. is hypoplastic or aplastic. It can be cut, if necessary.

The frontobasal segment of Falx is small, as small as the subdural route along Falx, until the arachnoid fold is reached which encloses the edge of Falx. The arachnoid fold must be incised along the edge of Falx. Now the interhemispheric subarachnoid space is opened. The following interhemispheric subarachnoid route is longer than the subdural route, until Lamina terminalis, the anterior wall of the 3rd ventricle, is reached.

Splitting of Lamina terminalis (b in Fig. 16) is limited by Chiasma and by Commissura anterior:
– The anterior wall of Recessus opticus is built by Lamina terminalis. Incision should be stopped before Recessus opticus is reached
– Commissura anterior is the inferior limit area of the Columnae-fornicis-For. interventriculare-complex.
  An incision of this area might result in damage of psychological functions.

Details (Figs. 17 to 18)

1. Comparison of translaminar and transforaminal approaches (Fig. 17)

Translaminar approaches are not as common as transforaminal approaches. Therefore the different anatomical aspects for surgery are described:

– Subdural route along Falx
  Translaminar: Gaps of Falx may revail adhesions of both frontal hemispheres
  Transforaminal: Rare

– Subarachnoidal route between the hemispheres

Translaminar: The subarachnoid route is long. Gyri of both hemispheres are bulging against each other. Now the routes present bended courses, containing numerous arachnoid trabeculae and adhesions
Transforaminal: Subarachnoid route short. Gyri of both hemispheres are flattened, not bulging.

– Opening of the 3rd ventricle
Translaminar: Narrow, less variable approaches
Incision of Lamina terminalis is problematic, because Allocortex is endangered, especially Area subcallosa
The hypothalamic vessels are endangered, too. Numerous perforating arteries are originating from A2, A.communicans ant., and from A. corporis callosi mediana (Yasargil's anterior hypothalamic artery).
Transforaminal: Wide variability for interhemispheric routes. Defining of the midline is problematic: Danger for a contralateral opening of the lateral ventricle with endangering of Columnae fornicis. Danger for the allocortical lateral striae of Corpus callosum and of the basal segment of Gyrus cinguli
Columna fornicis encloses the interventricular foramen and may be endangered by transforaminal approaches

2. Surgical aspects of variants of Lamina terminalis (Fig. 18)

Six types of Lamina terminalis were selected from MRTs of normal individuals. These types should be considered at splitting of Lamina terminalis, because the orientation may be difficult, regarding the narrow approaches in the depth

Intraventricular target areas (Figs. 19 and 20)

A straight view through the surgically fenestrated Lamina terminalis presents the posterior outline of the 3rd ventricle. It may be hindered by the variable or inconstant Adhaesio interthalamica. It may be transsected, if necessary.
Plexus can be moved on the side.
The view to the floor of the 3rd ventricle is distorted.
Using a flexible endoscope, this distortion can be avoided. Using the endoscope, all details can be presented in sectional enlargements. These presentations may be combined in a common panorama (Fig. 19 B). Fig. 20 presents the distorted outline of the ventricle by a straight view, using a microscope or a not straight endoscope.

Approaches transcrossing Foramen interventriculare (Monroi) – transforaminal approaches – (Figs. 21 to 30)

Principles of surgical approaches (Fig. 21)

Approaches transcrossing the interhemispheric space in the area of Bregma or anterior from it. After the favorable subdural route and the incision of the arachnoid fold at the edge of Falx, Cisterna corporis callosi is present immediately after separating the Gyri cinguli from each other. Before Corpus callosum is incised in a sagittal direction, Aa. pericallosae and its branches must be dissected and shifted aside. One or several midline crossing branches (for feeding the contralateral hemisphre, Marino et al 1975) should be carefully loosened and shifted, if it hinders the approach.
Danger of contralateral encephalomalazia!

Corpus callosum should be incised close to the midline, but lateral from the insertion line of Septum pellucidum. If the incision is done until the lateral ventricle is opened, then several subependymal veins would be cut, because these veins are running in a transverse direction into the roof of the lateral ventricle. The sagittal direction of the incision should be turned in a transversal direction, before the ventricular roof is opened. After this, the lateral ventricle can be inspected and the plexus may be used for a landmark: At its anterior end the interventricular foramen can be identified.

Details (Figs. 22 to 28)

1. Defining of the routes of approaches (Fig. 22 to 24)

Bregma, Foramen interventriculare, and Corpora mamillaria are located on one straight line (Fig. 22). But this may be only one of numerous routes which can be used for surgical approaches along the long-extended interhemisphreic space (Fig. 23). This is existing in contrast to transcerebral approaches, which are not to be discussed here.

But the numerous routes in midline approaches are restricted by bridging veins (Fig. 24)

2. Incision of Corpus callosum (Fig. 25)

The laterally located main portion of allocortical ("limbic") striae must be preserved during surgery for avoiding postoperative psychological deficits. This lateral bundle of striae is enclosed by the basal segment of Gyrus cinguli, dorsally from the lateral edge of Cisterna corporis callosi. All striae are continuations of Area dentata and Hippocampus, included the fine Striae corporis callosi.

A further problem of surgery may be the confusion of the right and left lateral ventricle by an incorrect incision of Corpus callosum.

The transversal subependymal veins of the roof of the lateral ventricle should be preserved, if possible.

Technical aspects of the incision of Corpus callosum

Brain shifting to one side, by spatula or sucker, e.g., may deviate the lateral ventricles, especially Septum pellucidum, against the homolateral side (This effect is reduced by using an endoscope). After brain shifting, an incision of Corpus callosum seems to be located ipsilateral. After such an error, the contralateral ventricle may be opened. This event can be avoided, if the incision is located close to the edge of Cisterna corporis callosi after reclination of the brain. The cingular striae are located at the level of the incision, but dorsal from it. Multiple fine fibers connect Striae corporis callosi and cingular striae in the area of incision of Corpus callosum. These fibers may be used for defining the location of incision.

Now the allocortical fibers of Gyrus cinguli and its numerous connections with Meso- and Neocortex of the fronto-parietal lobes are preserved. The ipsilateral ventricle can be opened.

For preservation of subependymal veins see Fig. 25 D and D'

For anatomical details of the limbic striae see H Stephan in 1975

3. 3rd ventricle and adjacent structures – endoscopical aspects – (Figs. 26 and 27)

Endoscopical topographies are sectional enlarged presentations, more than microsurgical topographies. So the spatial imagination may be supported by an overview of the intra- and extraventricular structures, which may be compared with the typical details.

This is less problematic at approximately horizontal approaches (translamellar and supracerebellar). Here many structures are presented by a straight view. For transforaminal and retroforaminal approaches a flexible endoscopy is necessary.

For the spatial imagination it is useful to compare the relief of the wall of the 3rd ventricle with adjacent structures in MRTs.

It is possible to compare the shape of a land-map with the shape of a sea-map. The outlines of the continents and the outlines of the oceans are identic, but not identic for the mental imagination. The mind sees only shapes, not outlines. The shapes of continents are seen, or the shapes of oceans, but not simultaneously both. A comparison of both avoids errors defining of proportions. These aspects are well known especially by painters, which learn it during their professional training.

Extra- and intraventricular target areas (Figs. 28 to 30)

The topography of the dorsal surface of the anterior and middle segment of Corpus callosum should be considered. The variable and narow topographical conditions of this area are shown in Fig. 28. After this, presentation of the lateral ventricle and location of the interventricular foramen is not problematic. The final problem is orientation in the 3rd ventricle transcrossing a wide or narrow interventricular foramen (Figs. 29 and 30).

If the interventricular foramen is masked by a space occupying lesion, e.g., it may be defined by following the plexus in the depth. Here the foramen is overlapped by a bulging and flattening of Columna fornicis. A typical example is a colloid cyst, which not always can be evacuated by a stereotactic puncture.

Approaches transpassing Fissura transversa – retroforaminal approaches – (Figs. 31 to 36)

Principles of surgical approaches (Fig. 31)

Interhemispheric routes and incision of Corpus callosum are similar to the transforaminal routes. But they are performed posterior from Foramen interventriculare. The lateral ventricle is opened as described for transforaminal routes. Depending on the location of the target area in the anterior or in the posterior segment of the 3rd ventricle, the ipsilateral layer of Septum pellucidum will be incised in an axial direction for opening of Cavum septi pellucidi. It will be spread. Now both layers of the Septum will be spread, until the bottom of Cavum septi pellucidi is reached. This bottom is the thin-walled connection of both Fornices. By spreading of the forceps this interfornical connection is easy to split. After this, Fissura transversa is opened. The inner cerebral veins are present, enclosed by Velum interpositum. The veins are bulging against the lumen of Fissura transversa. Between the inner cerebral veins, Velum interpositum can be split in a sagittal direction. Or it may be split lateral from it, if this is more favorable. The medial group of fine choroid arteries can be moved aside. These arteries present a parallel running without transversal connections. After incision and splitting of Velum interpositum the 3rd ventricle is opened.

Details (Figs. 32 to 36)

1. Avoiding bridging veins (Fig. 32)

There is the same problem as in transforaminal approaches.

2. Avoiding damage of a prefixed Fornix (Figs. 33 and 34)

Insertion of Fornix at Corpus callosum is located rostrally from the usual location, together with the posterior limit of Septum pellucidum. Surgical routes transpassing Cavum septi pellucidi are only possible in the shortened segment between Foramen interventriculare and the prepositioned Fornix. A widening of the approach in an anterior direction is normally blocked by the posterior wall of Foramen interventriculare, which is crossed over by V. thalamostriata, enclosed by plexus.

Often the posterior end of Cavum septi pellucidi is a little widened (Fig. 33 B), in normal conditions and at prefixed Fornices. This is favorable for interfornical splitting. Another favorable aspect at prefixed Fornix is the widening of Commissura fornicis. Anterior from the inferior surface of Splenium the commissure is wide enough for splitting of Corpus callosum and Commissura fornicis without endangering Crura fornicis. Before surgery this can be proved by MRT. Normally, Commissura fornicis is small and both Crura fornicis are endangered by splitting of Corpus callosum without an exact defining of the midline.

The midline is defined after splitting of Commissura fornicis by regarding the inner cerebral veins. The opening of the dorsal wall of the 3rd ventricle can be performed as described for interfornical splitting.

3. Cavum Vergae (Fig. 35)

Cavum Vergae is a common variant, like the prefixed Fornix. This is the widened posterior segment of (the often common widened) Cavum septi pellucidi, based on the first description of Verga (1851). In 1981 Lang has given a detailed description. He added observations of openings of the lateral and of the basal wall of Cavum Vergae, which may connect Cavum Vergae and Atrium ventriculi, as well as Fissura transversa. He described these observations in contrast to the clinical observations. At numerous clinical observations, Cavum Vergae seems to be not connected with other CSF-spaces. Perhaps the SCF-fluid is obstructred by the numerous adhesions. But it cannot be understood, that communications of Cavum Vergae and the lateral ventricle at clinical findings are even not to be confirmed. Cavum Vergae is a favorable precondition for surgical approaches to the 3rd ventricle. Using the widened and voluminous Cavum Vergae, splitting of Septum pellucidum for opening of Cavum septi pellucidi/Cavum Vergae is not problematic. Both Fornices are distant from each other. Interfornical splitting of the ground of Cavum septi pellucidi/Cavum Vergae does not endanger Fornices.

The midline may be defined using the location of the inner cerebral veins.

But there exists a further topographical problem. Cavum Vergae and Splenium are widened in a far posterior direction. They are overlapping Cisterna tecti and its neighboring tectal structures much more than in normal conditions. For sugery it is important to define the posterior dorsal limit point of the 3rd ventricle. This point may be defined by Commissura posterior, using a median sagittal slice of MRT and mapping this by neuronavigation. During surgery, Corpus pineale may be used as landmark, if neuronavigation is not available.

4. V. ventriculi lat. directa (Fig. 36)

This variant of veins is a favorable precondition for a surgical widening of Foramen interventriculare (Monroi) in a posterior direction. V. ventriculi lat. directa is a substitute for V. thalamostriata. V. ventriculi lat. directa is located far posterior from Foramen interventriculare. The posterior wall of the foramen does not contain V. thalamostriata. The wall can be incised without interruption of an important vein. Only the fine V. septi pellucidi is present. It can be shifted aside. Now Foramen interventriculare is widened in a posterior direction.

Supracerebellar approaches for the 3rd ventricle and surrounding structures (Krause-Yasargil) (Figs. 37 to 47)

Principles of surgical approaches (Fig. 37)

The principles of trepanation and of the dural opening are following the same principles as in supratentorial midline approaches for the 3rd ventricle: Trepanation is performed up to the sinus (here: Sinus transversus) is visible. The dural incision is stopped at the margin of the sinus. In contrast to supratentorial approaches, no bridging veins are underlying the inside of the dura. Now the dural flap can be elevated.

The subdural route is started between the dural doubling (here: Tentorium), and the outer arachnoid layer of the dorsal cerebellar surface. This part of the route is interrupted at the tentorial edge, which is enclosed by the transit of the outer arachnoid layer from its infratentorial to its supratentorial portion. This layer is extended after shifting the cerebellar surface with the outer arachnoid layer downwards.

The next step is the incision of this thickwalled and not transparent outer cerebello-tentorial arachnoid layer, which covers Cisternae ambientes and Cisterna tecti. Its adhesions with the galenic vein must be taken into consideration, studying MRT's (Fig. 12). The incision of Arachnoidea should be performed as basally as possible, at the anterior margin of Culmen. It begins with a small incision **lateral from the midline** (lateral from the galenic vein), which may be widened bilaterally in a horizontal direction.

After this, Cisternae are opened, and the difficult dissection of arachnoid trabeculae and arachnoid membranes and adhesions may be done. Vessels and – if necessary – N. trochlearis, can be loosened and – if necessary – shifted aside. Cave Corpus pineale, because its adjacent structures are connected with the surrounding structures of Aquaeductus!
At last the area of Recessus suprapinealis is reached. Its wall is translucent and may rupture by surgical manipulations before it is identified.
Now two different target areas may be presented:
– The third ventricle
– Fissura transversa along the galenic vein, then dorsal from it

Details (Figs. 38 to 42)

1. Positioning on the operating table (Fig. 38)

The narrow routes and the manipulations in the depth as well as intracranial pressure make a sitting position of the patient more favorable. Fig. 38 presents landmarks which can be used, if a horizontal view is wanted by the surgeon. But this may be variable, depending on the variable technical methods which can be used.

2. Avoiding bridging veins (Fig. 39)

The bridging veins of the dorsal surface of Cerebellum are connected to Tentorium close to Sinus transversus or to this sinus, but without a connection to the dorsal dura.

A typical bundle of thick veins is located medially.

Therefore Yasargil stated the approaches lateral from these veins*. A diagonal route in a medial direction to Culmen cerebelli was preferred. Yasargil* modified this route depending on variants of the bridging veins.

In the midline some fine bridging veins are running from Vermis sup. to Sinus rectus. After their cutting Culmen is sinking down, and the outer arachnoid layer of Cisterna tecti can be incised.

3. Avoiding V. magna Galeni and adjacent structures of Aquaeductus (Figs. 40 to 42)

The transitional area of the galenic vein and of Sinus rectus at the inferior surface of the tentorial edge may be dark in color. Between fine transversal gaps of the fibrous tissue, veins may be recognizable. Below this area the galenic vein is masked by the thick-walled outer arachnoid layer of Cisterna tecti. The close relationship of the inferior loop of galenic vein and Corpus pineale/Tectum can be illustrated by a median-sagittal slice in MRT (Fig. 12). Typically, the galenic vein is adherent to the outer arachnoid layer of Cisterna tecti and to the Recessus-suprapinealis-Corpus pineale complex. For preservation of the vein, the incision of the outer arachnoid layer should be started basally, immediately close and parallel to the anterior margin of Culmen cerebelli. A short and stepwise incision should be performed to avoid injuring the galenic vein. Unexpected bleeding is easy to control by standard surgical and anesthesiological methods. After this, the incision can be extended so that Cisterna ambiens is bilaterally visible, if necessary.

The next surgical step is the preservation of vessels in Cisterna tecti and the preservation of cerebral structures adjacent to Aquaeductus and its connections with Corpus pineale.

Veins are located close to the midline. A bundle of thick-calibrated anterior cerebellar veins and supraculminal veins are entering the inferior loop of the galenic vein, as well as the mostly fine bilateral tectal veins, which are converging to the midline before entering the thick veins or the galenic vein. Most of the veins are overlying the choroid arteries lateral to Tectum. Some fine branches are feeding Tectum and Corpus pineale.

Sometimes, vessels can be easily shifted aside. But often multiple arachnoid trabeculae and membranes and adhesions must be moved, and Corpus pineale, Habenula, Thalamus and the other structures, which are located close to the entrance of the Aquaeductus, are presented intact. Even with careful manipulation, usually CSF flaks out of the incised or spontaneous ruptured Recessus suprapinealis of the 3rd ventricle.

Target areas of the 3rd ventricle and of Fissura transversa (Figs. 43 to 47)

The surgical route to target areas around the 3rd ventricle and Fissura transversa requires crossing the cisternal space between Corpus pineale and the galenic vein. In this route, Recessus suprapinealis is interposed. This area is richly vascularized, and it contains a variable number of arachnoid trabeculae and adhesions. These arachnoid structures build solid connections between the galenic vein and Corpus pineale, enclosing

---

* Personal communication

the recessus. If loosening of the adhesions is incomplete, the connections of Corpus pineale with its adjacent cerebral structures may be injured:
– Habenula and its peduncle at Corpus pineale
– Habenula and its connection to Thalamus
– Commissura habenularum and its connection to Corpus pineale and to Commissura posterior
– subependymal gray matter of all these structures enclosing the area of entrance of Aquaeductus. Damage of these areas may lead to deficits of vegetative functions and of alertness.

After insertion of the endoscope and cutting of Adhaesio interthalamica (if necessary), the following structures can be distinguished
– Structures of the anterior area of the 3rd ventricle
– Structures of the roof of the 3rd ventricle
– Structures of the floor of the 3rd ventricle
– Structures of the posterior area of the 3rd ventricle

Structures of the anterior area of the 3rd ventricle
– Both Columnae fornicis
– Commissura anterior between Columnae fornicis, before Columnae are penetrating the wall of the ventricle (transition of Pars libera and Pars tecta fornicis)
– A trigonal shaped fovea, above Commissura anterior.
  Its shape is defined by Commissura anterior and Columnae fornicis. A median-sagittal slice of MRT is presenting this fovea: It is the area of the connections of Commissura anterior, Rostrum corporis callosi, Septum pellucidum, Columnae fornicis. Foramen interventriculare (Monroi) is located close to it and superior-posterior from it.

– Foramen interventriculare (Monroi)
Its medial-anterior margin is formed by Columnae fornicis
Its lateral margin is formed by Tuberculum ant. thalami (containing Nucleus ant. thalami), and the transitional area of Pars libera fornicis to Pars tecta fornicis

Structures of the roof of the 3rd ventricle:
– Plexus chorioideus, which becomes smaller and ends, before Recessus suprapinealis is reached.
– Velum interpositum, the origin of the plexus, is connectred with Striae medullares thalami by Taeniae thalami, before it enlarges at the surface of the Thalami.
– The inner cerebral veins, which are enclosed by Velum interpositum. The location of the junction of Vv.cerebri intt. and the length of V. magna Galeni are variable. The junction may be located posterior or anterior from Recessus suprapinealis.
  This is recognizable better on axial slices of MRTs than by anatomical cadaver dissections

Structures of the floor of the 3rd ventricle:
– Recessus opticus. Its anterior wall is the extension of Lamina terminalis in a basal direction. Its posterior wall is identic with the dorsal segment of Chiasma. This segment of Chiasma is interposed between Recessus opticus and Recessus infundibuli
– Recessus infundibuli. Its surrounding structures are Infundibulum and, at its extraventricular surface, Tuber cinereum.
– Corpora mamillaria are bulge against the ventricular lumen. These landmarks may be flattened by hydrocephalus. But they are to be identified by a typical bilateral bundle of subependymal fine vessels, which are especially feeding the gray matter of the inner segments of Corpora mamillaria. Behind Corpora mamillaria, the wall of the ven-

tricle becomes thickened, before Aquaeductus is reached. This segment represents the upper area of Tectum. Sulcus prae- and Recessus postmamillaris sometimes cannot be identified.

The fibers of Crura cerebri are located beside Corpora mamillaria. Arteries in these areas are coming from Substantia perforata post. (perforators).

Structures of the posterior area of the 3rd ventricle:
– Entrance of Aquaeductus. This is the border of Tegmentum and of Tectum mesencephali, surrounded by Griseum centrale (Substantia grisea centralis mesencephali). Its roof is bulging:
– Commissura posterior. Commissura habenularum and the commissure of both Colliculi superiores are adjacent to this commissure. All these structures are located in the roof of the entrance of Aquaeductus. Commissura posterior is bulging against the ventricle between Aquaeductus and Recessus pinealis

The structures of the ventricular floor are better visible by a transforaminal and, if necessary, by a retroforaminal approach, than by a supracerebellar approach.
The posterior wall can be better identified by a translaminar route than by supracerebellar routes. All structures are visible using a flexible endoscope.

Addendum
Target area Fissura transversa

The visualization of Fissura tranversa and surrounding structures is still difficult. Fissura transversa is a rare target area. The choroid membrane between the 3rd ventricle and Fissura transversa made approaches difficult in the past. In the nineteenth century, it was already called Velum interpositum as it is today. In the nomenclature of Basel (1896) it was called "Tela chorioidea ventriculi tertii". But the roof with plexus of the 3rd ventricle is only a small segment of it. In the twentieth century, the term "Tela chorioidea" was considered inappropiate because its dorsal surface is located not in a ventricular lumen, but in Fissura transversa, which is a cisternal CSF-space. Now it is well known that Velum interpositum is a plexus, indeed, with production of CSF into the ventricular lumen (3rd ventricle) and into a cisternal space (Fissura transversa).

Fissura transversa can be approached by the same supracerebellar route as used for the approach to the 3rd ventricle until Recessus suprapinealis is reached. When CSF leaks through the opened Recessus suprapinealis, the 3rd ventricle will collapse. Now the galenic vein can be freed from adhesions. These adhesions fill the transitional area of Cisterna tecti, Cisterna Galeni, and of Fissura transversa. After loosening of the adhesions, Fissura transversa is opened. By a straight view its posterior segment is visible. Visualization of the anterior segment is obstructed by the bulging of Thalami in a dorsal direction.
All segments of the fissure can be visualized by a flexible endoscope.
The following structures can be distinguished
– the floor of Fissura transversa
– the roof of Fissura transversa
– the lateral connection of the floor and the roof

Outline of the floor of Fissura transversa:
– Velum interpositum represents the floor of Fissura transversa. The velum covers Vv. cerebri intt. and the anterior segment of the galenic vein. This segment is variable, as seen in axial slices of MRTs. Striae and Taeniae thalami connect the plexus of the 3rd

ventricle with the dorsomedial margin of Thalamus. These can be identified at a view into Fissura transversa. The triangular-shaped floor of Fissura transversa is laterally limited by a rim, Fissura chorioidea. Taenia chorioidea and Taenia fornicis are connected in this area. The plexus protrudes into the lateral ventricle. Both Taenia chorioidea and Taenia fornicis can be identified at a view into Fissura transversa. Manipulations in this area may result in occult intraventricular bleeding from the plexus of the lateral ventricle. Cave! Fine medial bundles of the choroid arteries are running parallel to the inner cerebral veins. The lateral bundles are diverging and penetrate Fissura chorioidea. They are not feeding exclusively the plexus of the lateral ventricle. Some branches penetrate Fissura chorioidea and the dorsal surface of Thalamus. Veins are more variable. A dorsal thalamic vein often penetrates the medial surface of Thalamus close to Taenia thalami and enters V. cerebri int.. This dorsal thalamic vein is a bilateral vessel. Sometimes the thick-calibrated V. ventricularis inf. is running from its superior end into a transversal direction. For V. ventriculi lat. directa see Fig. 36.

Outline of the roof of Fissura transversa:
– The roof is formed by Corpora fornicis and their continuations, the Crura fornicis, and of Commissura fornicis. The transitional area of Corpora and Crura fornicis is the top of the triangular-shaped Commissura fornicis, which is enclosed by approximately parallel triangular shape of the Fornices. The tip of Commissura fornicis is the level of the invisible posterior end of Septum pellucidum and the other side of Fornices. The limits of Fornices are well defined, contrary to the ventricular limit. A view into Fissura transversa shows a bulging of Fornices against the lumen of the fissure. Commissura fornicis is excavated in a dorsal direction. Both, Crura fornices and Commissura fornicis, join Corpus callosum on the other side. Anterior from it, Corpora fornicis join each other in the midline. They are separated to each other by a rim. On the other side of this rim ends Cavum septi pellucidi. The rostral tip of the triangular-shaped Fissura transversa is formed by the cisternal surface of the posterior wall of both Foramina interventricularia (Monroi). Plexus and the beginning of the inner cerebral veins may be seen, enclosed by the leptomeninges of Fissura transversa. On the intraventricular surface of the posterior wall of the intraventricular foramina the wall is enclosed by Ependyma.
  Between floor and roof of Fissura transversa some fine vessels or adhesions may be extended, which usually do not cause any problem during surgery, except in pathological findings, such as AVMs.

The lateral connection of the floor and roof of Fissura transversa:
– These lines correspond to Fissura chorioidea at each lateral border of Fissura transversa. In Fissura chorioidea Taenia fornicis and Taenia chorioidea connect, and insert into the Plexus chorioideus of the lateral ventricle. Taenia fornicis normally contains no fine vessels, but the medial septal veins and the medial atrial veins cross this Taenia before entering Taenia chorioidea – velum interpositum-complex and its veins.
  Taenia chorioidea is richly vascularized. Lateral atrial veins are connected to the inner cerebral veins, crossing Taenia chorioidea, as well as variants of the inferior ventricular vein, which can be seen at the floor of Fissura transversa, enclosed by Velum interpositum. These vessels must be spared at surgery of meningiomas, cavernomas, plexus papillomas, AVMs and other pathological findings, which may be enclosed by Fissura transversa. Space-occupying lesions and vascular malformations of Cisterna tecti, of the lateral ventricle or of Corpus callosum may involve Fissura transversa. The description of AVMs of Corpus callosum by Yasargil is well known. Here an exact presentation of the surgical problems of the area of Fissura transversa is given.

Fig. 1

Overview of surgical approaches

a	Translaminar approaches
b	Transforaminal approaches
c	Retroforaminal approaches
d	Supracerebellar approaches

c and *d*   Combined approaches for Fissura transversa and for the 3rd ventricle

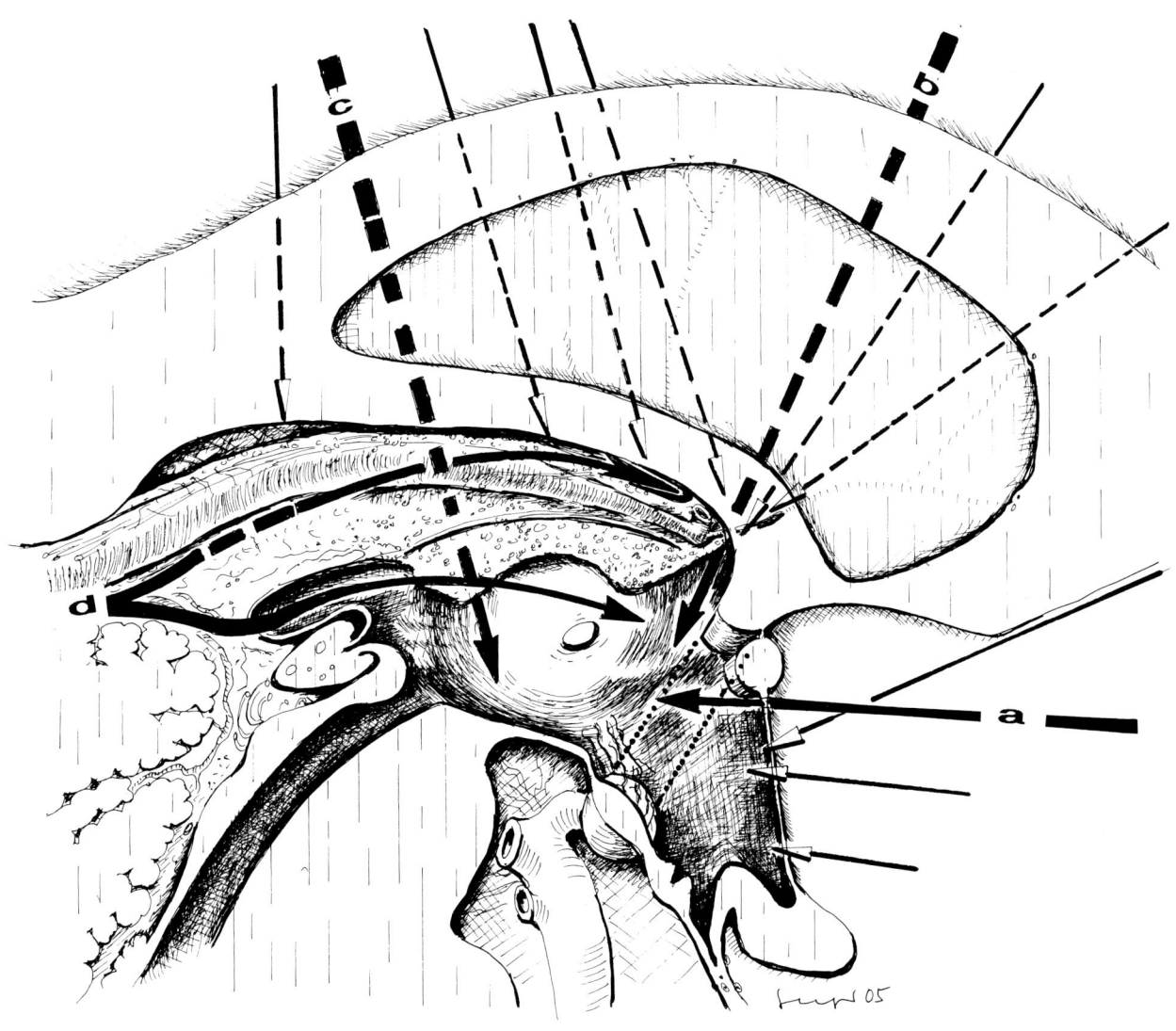

ANATOMICAL BACKGROUND (Figs. 2 to 15)

Fig. 2

Overview

A   3rd ventricle according to an historical anatomical cast (Retzius 1900)
B   As A. Surrounding structures of the 3rd ventricle are indicated

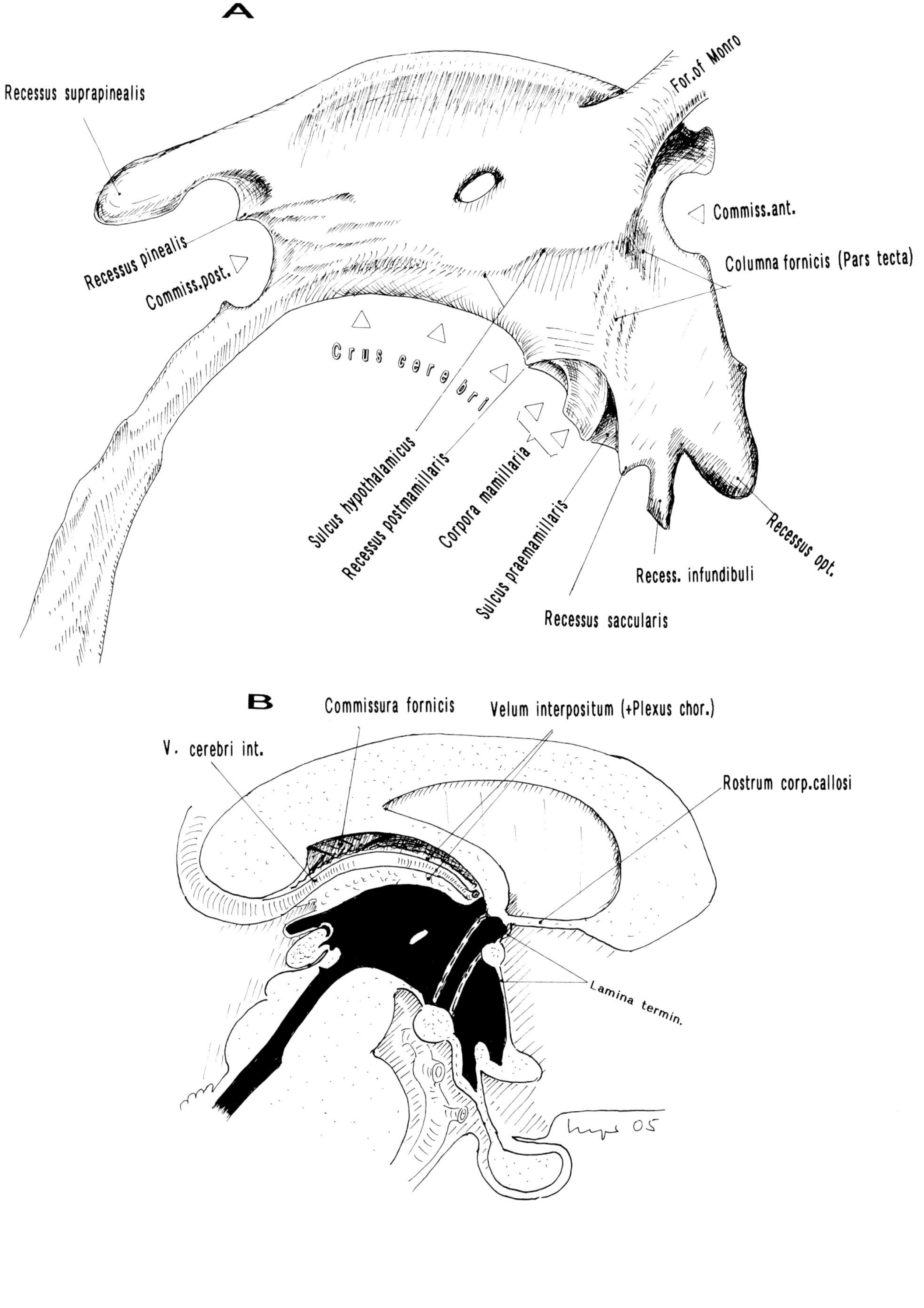

A

Recessus suprapinealis

For.of Monro

Recessus pinealis

Commiss.post. ◁

◁ Commiss.ant.

Columna fornicis (Pars tecta)

◁   △   ◁

Crus cerebri

△

◁

Sulcus hypothalamicus

Recessus postmamillaris

Corpora mamillaria

Sulcus praemamillaris

Recessus saccularis

Recess. infundibuli

Recessus opt.

B

Commissura fornicis

Velum interpositum (+Plexus chor.)

V. cerebri int.

Rostrum corp.callosi

Lamina termin.

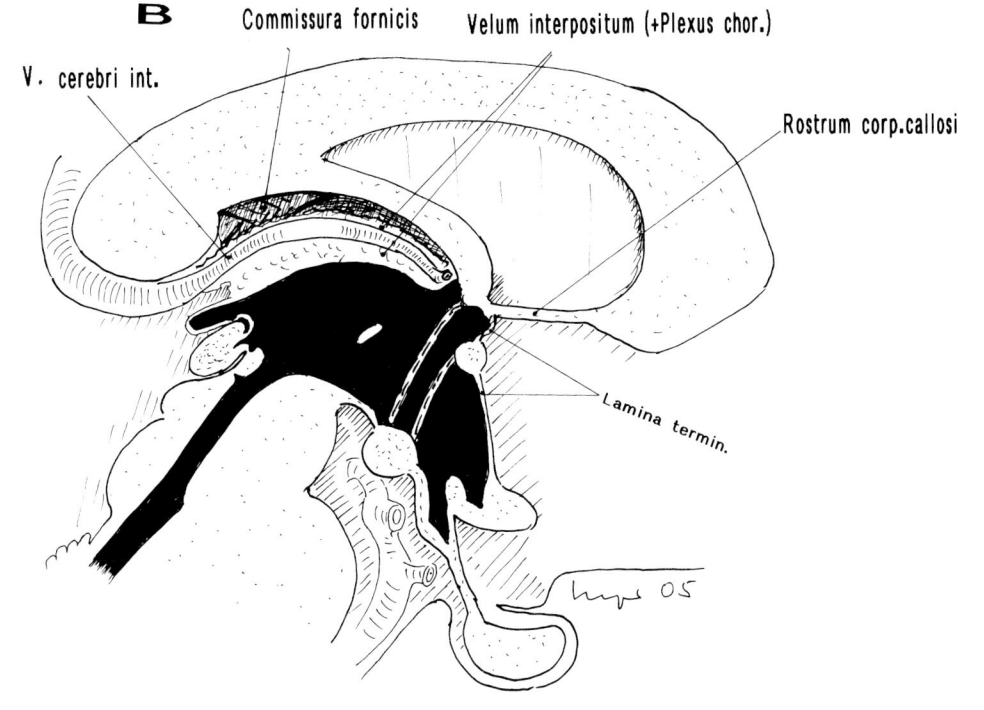

hupe 05

Details (Figs. 3 to 15)

Fig. 3

Anterior segment of the 3rd ventricle. Anatomical dissections

A   Sagittal presentation, overview
Note small perforating branches from A2/A. communicans ant.-t- and from A corporis callosi mediana ("anterior hypothalamic artery" of Yasargil –s-)

B   Coronal transection, schematical presentation
Plexus chorioideus, Velum interpositum, and Vv. cerebri intt. omitted
Note posterior surface of Columnae fornicis – anterior outline of Foramina interventricularia Monroi –a-

C   Asymmetrical shape of Columnae fornicis, as presented in coronal slices of MRT

C'   Asymetrical shape. This is a common finding presented in coronal slices of MRT

D   Asymmetrical shape. This is a common finding presented in coronal slices of MRT

D and **D'** Common variants of the Plexus chor. of the third ventricle

Abbreviations

a	For. interventriculare (Monroi)	*n*	Infundibulum
b	Vv. cerebri intt.	*o*	Chiasma
c	Fissura transversa cerebri	*p*	Recessus opt.
d	Columna(ae) fornicis, Pars libera	*q*	Commissura ant.
e	As d, Pars tecta	*r*	Lamina terminalis
f	Corpus mamillare	*s*	A. corporis callosi mediana
g	Recessus saccularis	*t*	A. communicans ant.
h	Sulcus praemamillaris	*u*	V. septi pellucidi
i	Recessus postmamillaris	*v*	Septum pellucidum
j	Thalamus	*w*	Velum interpositum, enclosing b
k	Sulcus hypothalamicus	*x*	Plexus chor.
l	Adhaesio interthalamica	*y*	Tuber cinereum
m	Recessus infundibuli	*z*	Gyrus rectus (and Area subcallosa)

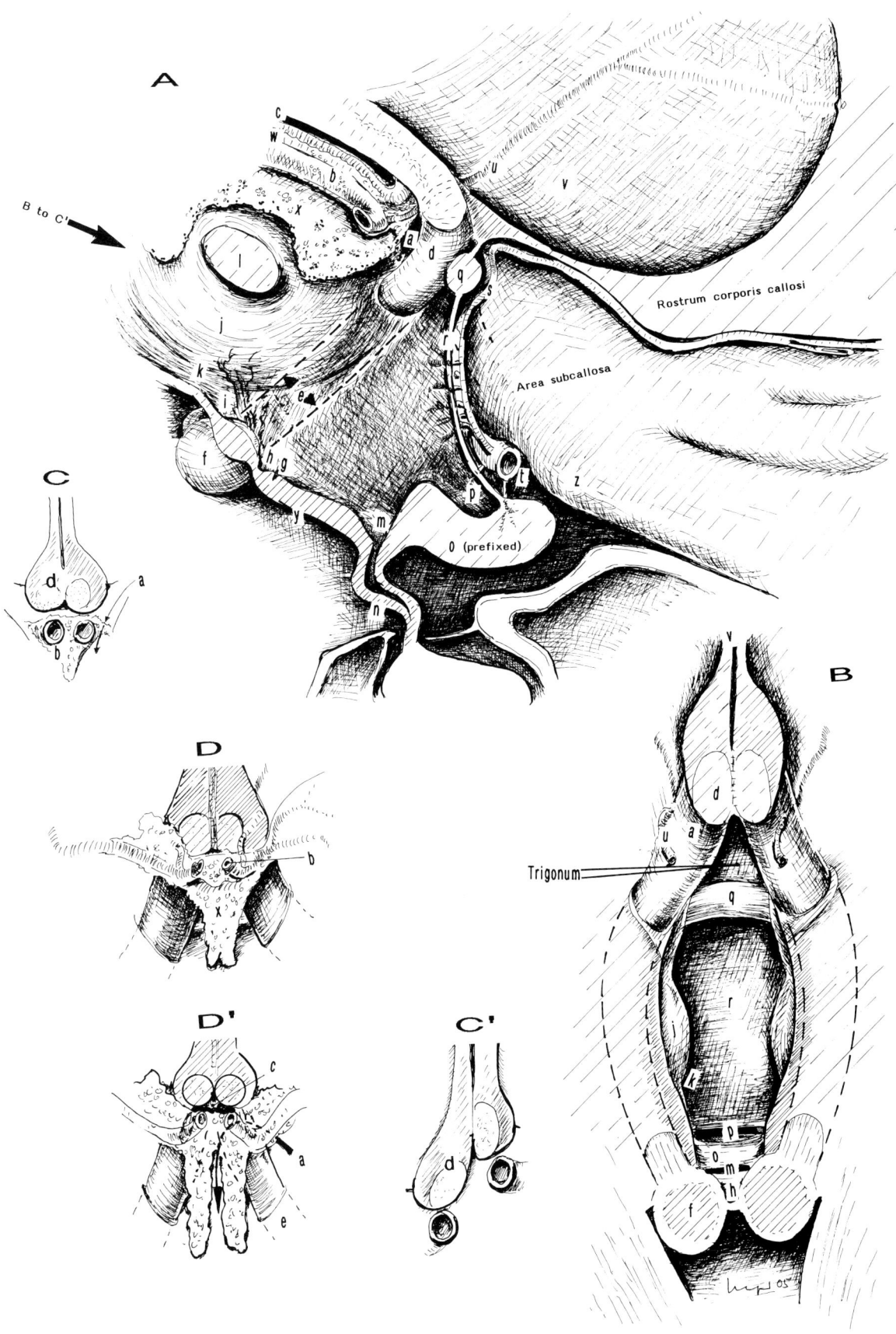

A

B to C'

Rostrum corporis callosi

Area subcallosa

0 (prefixed)

C

D

D'

C'

B

Trigonum

Fig. 4

Continuation of Fig. 3

3rd ventricle and its anterior adjacent structures, overview
Axial presentation of MRT, parallel to the intercommissural level

Abbreviations
a	Falx, inferior margin
b	fold of extern arachnoid layer, enclosing Falx
c	Sulcus cinguli
d	Gyrus anterior from Gyrus cinguli
e	Sulcus longitudinalis between both Gyri cinguli, anterior from Genu corp.call.
f	Striae of Gyrus cinguli
f'	Striae corporis callosi
g	as f, splitted
g'	as f', thickened bundles
h	Area subcallosa (allocortical)
i	as e, inferior from Rostrum corp.call.
j and *j'*	A2
j"	A. pericallosa
k	Commissura ant.
l	Columna fornicis, white bundle
l'	Columna fornicis, gray matter
m	Recessus opt.
n	Chiasma
o	Recessus infundibuli
p	Sulcus praemamillaris
p'	Recessus saccularis
q	Corpus mamillare
r	Commissura post.
r'	Aquaeductus (arrow)
r"	Recessus pinealis (arrow)
s	wall of Recessus suprapinealis
t	Corpus pineale
u	transition Genu-Rostrum
u'	posterior Rostrum fibers
v	A callosomarginalis

FIG. 4

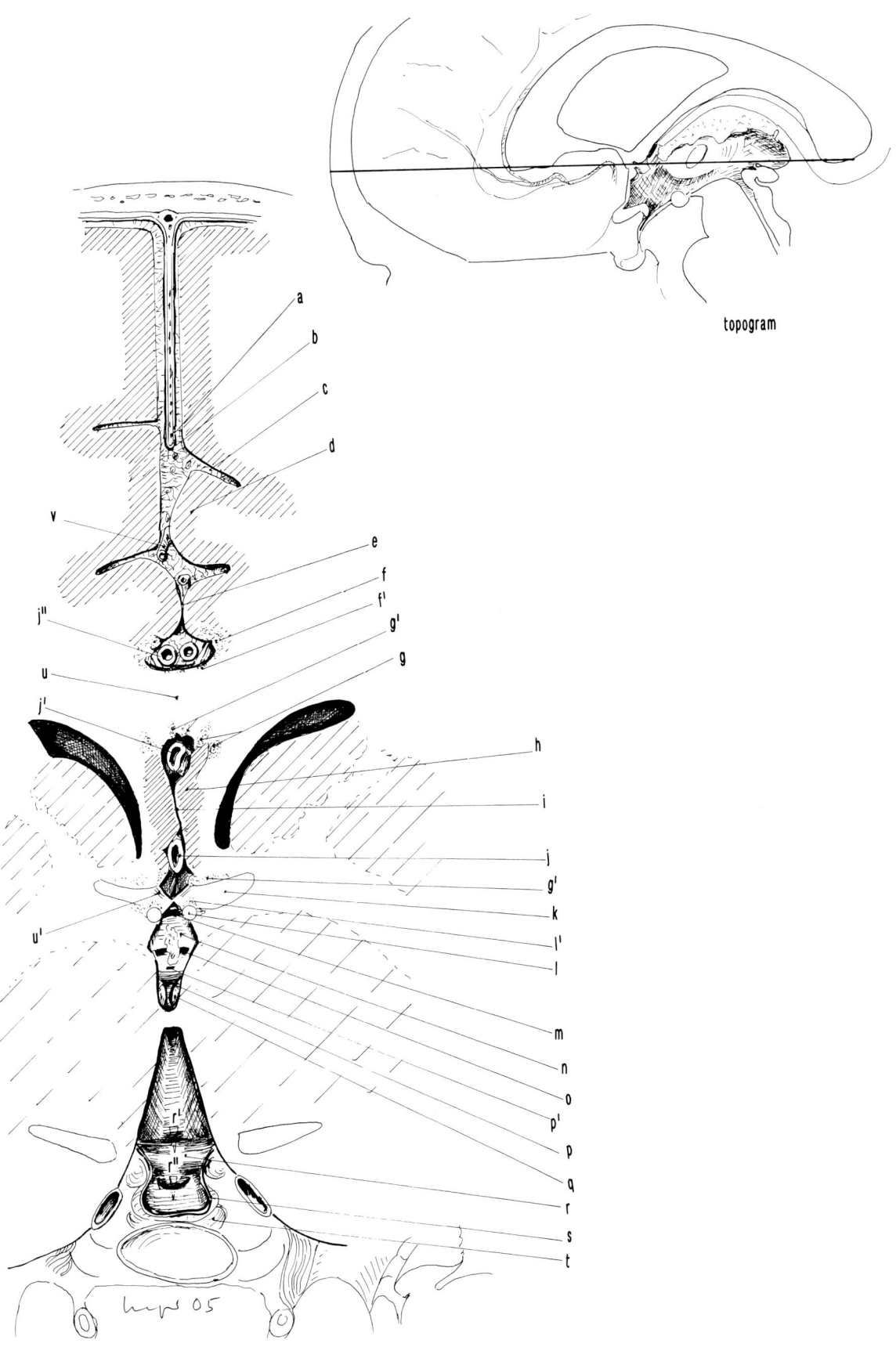

topogram

Fig. 5

3rd ventricle and its posterior adjacent structures, overview
Axial presentation of MRT, parallel to the intercommissural level

A   MRT according to Fig. 4
A'   Sectional enlargment of the anterior segment
A"   Sectional enlargment of the posterior segment, sagittal topogram for A

Abbreviations
a   Commissura ant.
b   Recessus opt.
c   Chiasma
d   Sulcus praemamillaris
e   Commissura post.
e'   Recessus pinealis
f   Recessus suprapinealis
g   V. basalis Rosenthal
g'   Rr. chorioidei postt.
h   V. magna Galeni
i   Columna fornicis
j   Plexus chorioideus
k   Recessus infundibuli
l   Thalamus
m   Adhaesio interthalamica
n   As 1
o   Habenula
p   Corpus pineale
q   Colliculus sup.
r   Colliculus inf.
s   N. IV
t   Splenium corporis callosi
u   A. cerebri post.
v   Lobulus centralis cerebelli
w   edge of Tentorium, enclosed by arachnoid fold
x   Tentorium
y   Culmen

FIG. 5

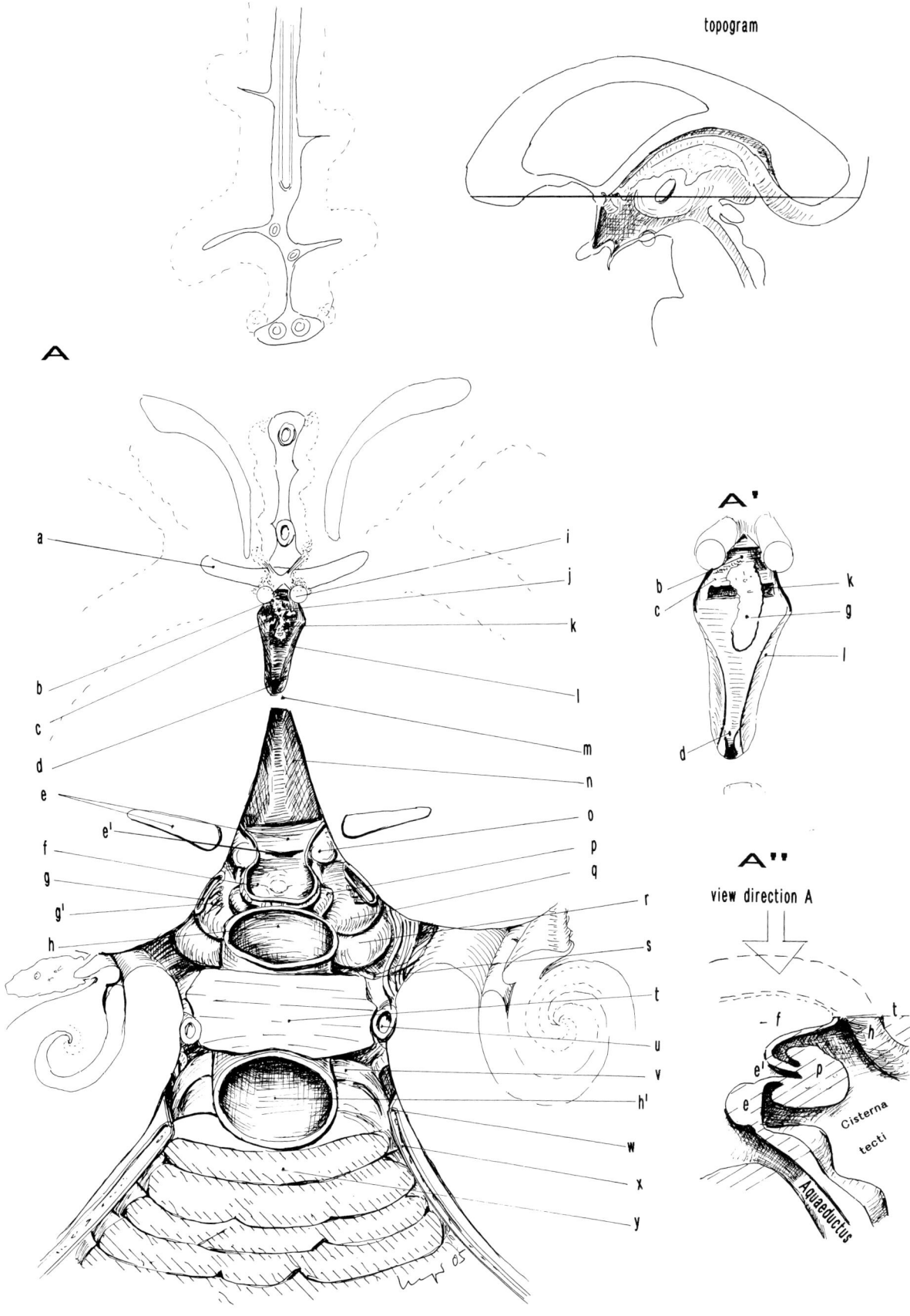

topogram

A

A'

A''

view direction A

Cisterna tecti

Aquaeductus

Fig. 6

Corpus callosum

MRTs (copies, simplified). Common findings

A   Genu corporis callosi thickened, Rostrum thinwalled

B   Middle segment of Corpus callosum thickened, Splenium bulging into a dorsal direction

C   Rostrum thickened. If it should be splitted at surgery, then Fornices and Commissura ant. may be endangered, if it would be mixed up with the thickwalled proximal located transition of Genu and Rostrum corporis callosi

D   Middle or posterior segment of Corpus callosum thinwalled

E   For comparison with C (and D)

FIG. 6

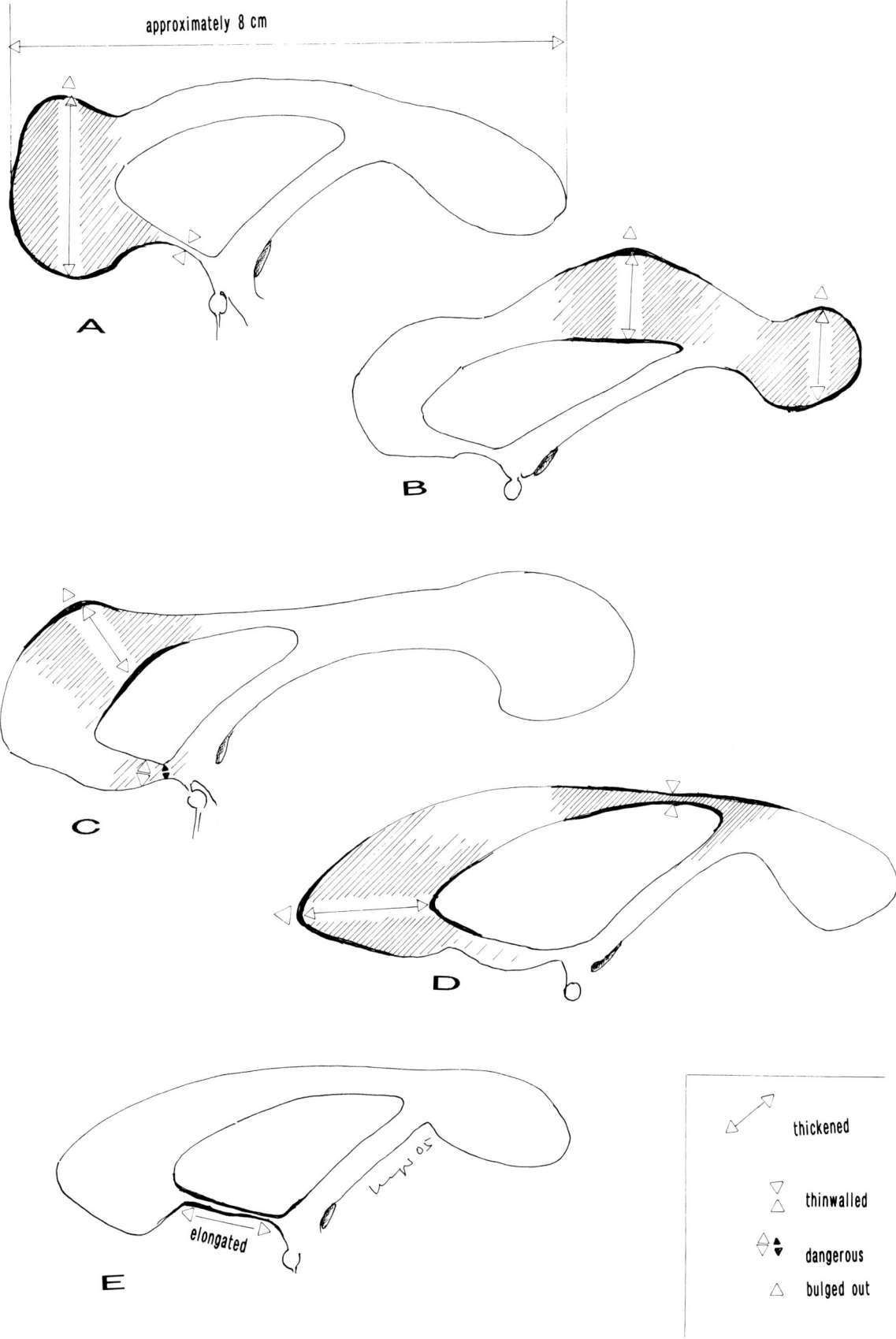

approximately 8 cm

A

B

C

D

E

elongated

thickened

thinwalled

dangerous

bulged out

Fig. 7

Addendum for Fig. 6

Rostrum corporis callosi and Lamina terminalis

Normal individuals, simplified presentations of MRTs
Landmark: Commissura ant. Intercommissural lines and vertical lines added

FIG. 7

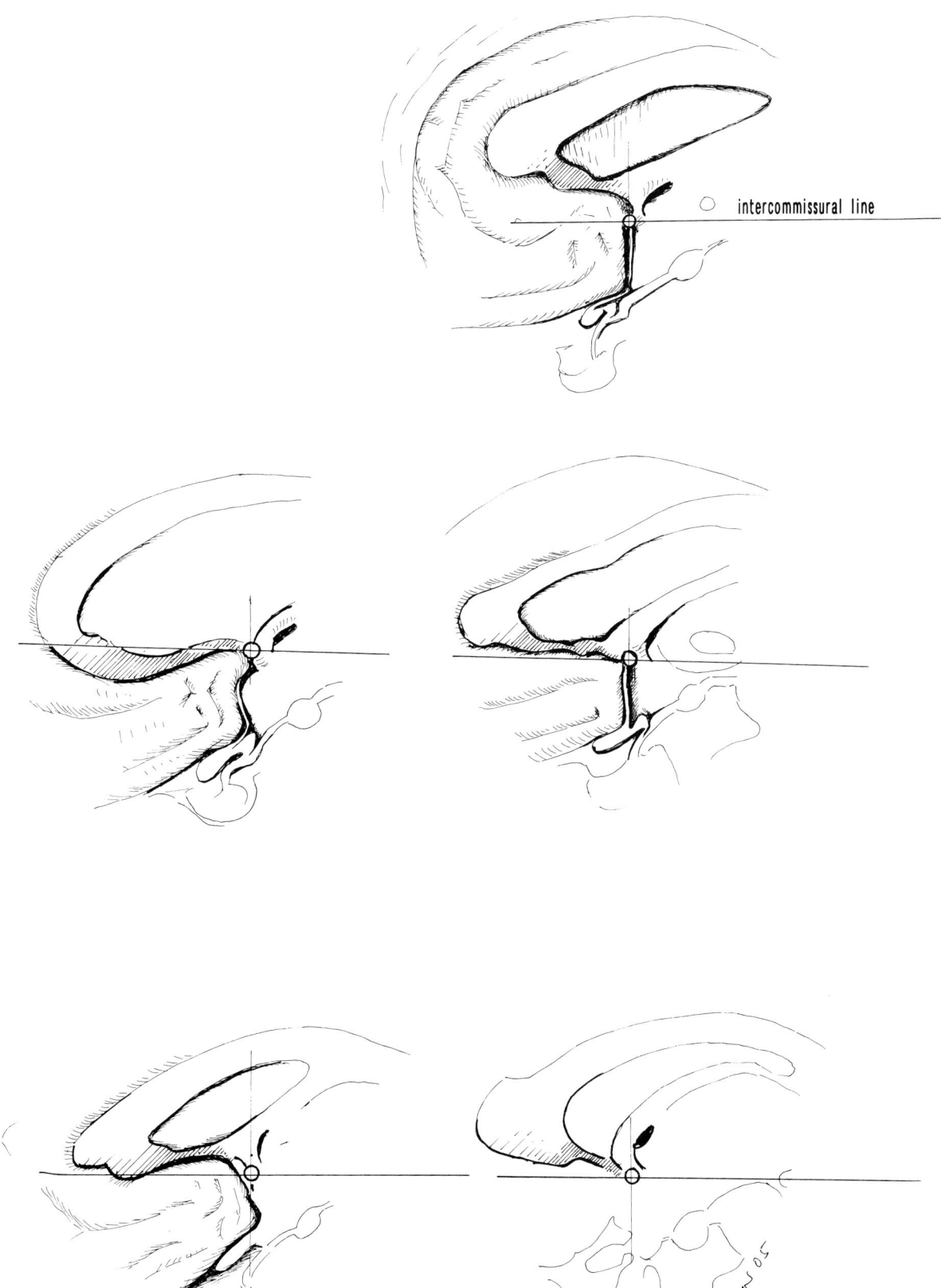

intercommissural line

Fig. 8

Callosodorsal and subcallosal Allocortex* according to Stephan (1975)

– Gyrus cinguli (mesocortical)
– Striae of Gyrus cinguli (allocortical)
– Medial and lateral Striae corporis callosi (allocortical)
– fine fibers connecting Striae corporis callosi (allocortical)
– fine fibers connecting Striae gyri cinguli and Striae latt. of Corpus callosum
   These fine fibers form the lateral rim of Cisterna corporis callosi
– Area subcallosa (mesocortical)
– Gyrus rectus (anterior segment neocortical, posterior segment meso- and allocortical)
– Trigonum olfactorium and its striae (allocortical)
   Stria medialis of Trigonum continues into the medial Striae corporis callosi
   Stria lat. of Trigonum continues into Corpus amygdaloides and Gyrus parahippo-
   campalis
– Commissura ant. (allocortical)

Definings according to Stephan (1975)
Allocortex: So-called "limbic" cortex
Mesocortex: Mixture of allo- and neocortical parts
Neocortex: Isocortex

_____

* Drawing according to Seeger (1978), modified

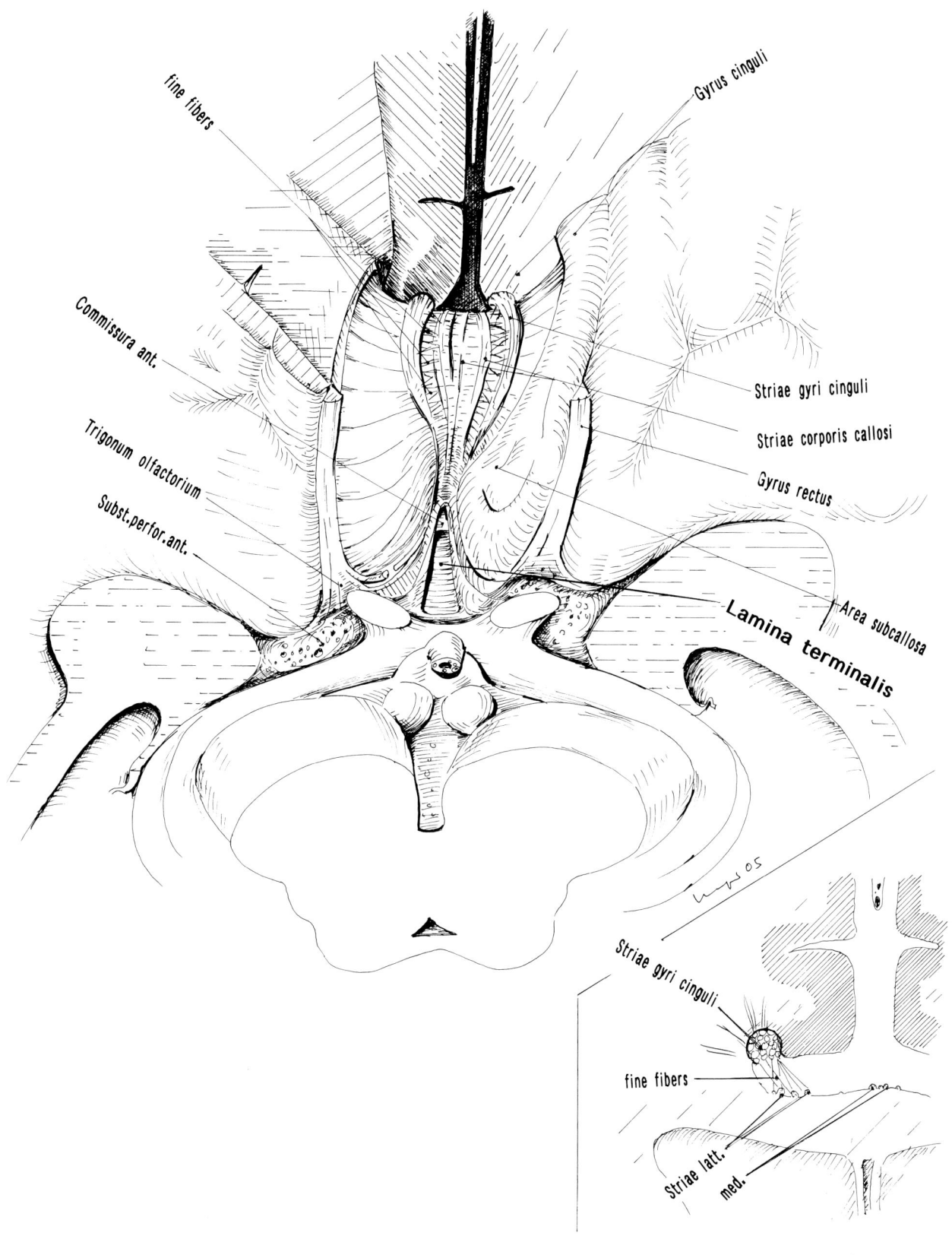

fine fibers

Gyrus cinguli

Commissura ant.

Trigonum olfactorium

Subst.perfor.ant.

Striae gyri cinguli

Striae corporis callosi

Gyrus rectus

Area subcallosa

Lamina terminalis

Striae gyri cinguli

fine fibers

Striae latt.

med.

Fornices (Figs. 9 to 11)

Fig. 9

Fornix and Septum pellucidum, common types. Anatomical sketches

A   Usual finding
Commissura fornicis –c- is interposed between the posterior end of Septum pellucidum and the anterior inferior limit of Splenium corporis callosi

B   Prefixed Fornices
The posterior end of Septum pellucidum and the anterior inferior limit of Splenium are located far away from each other
Commissura fornicis is enlarged (see –c- in B and B'')

C   Cavum Vergae
This cavum is a widened posterior segment of Cavum septi pellucidi, which is elongated in a posterior direction. Cavum Vergae is enclosed by a flattened Splenium. Commissura fornicis is widened and dislocated in a basal direction. The posterior area of the commissure is connected with the thinwalled anterior inferior end of Splenium. Defects of the lateral wall and of the floor of Cavum Vergae are typical findings (Lang). Its communication with Atrium ventriculi or with Fissura transversa may be inconstant

A' to C'' Coronal transections

Abbreviations
a   Septum pellucidum
a'   Cavum septi pellucidi
a''   Cavum Vergae
b   Columna fornicis
c   Commissura fornicis
d   Crus fornicis
e   Plexus chorioideus
f   Corpus callosum
g   Fissura transversa
h   Defects of the wall of Cavum Vergae
i   V. cerebri int.
j   V. magna (Galeni)
k   For. interventriculare (Monroi)

FIG. 9

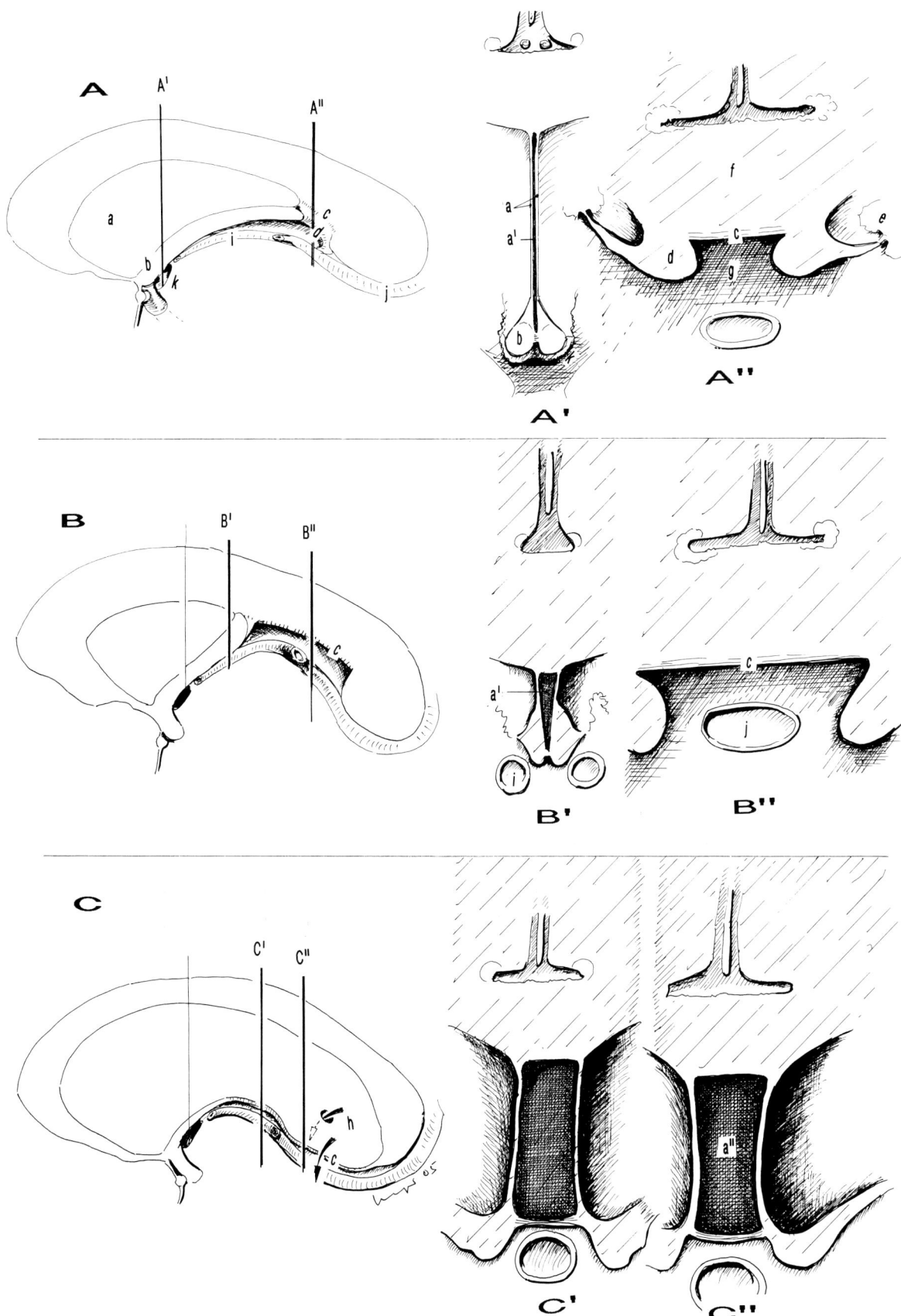

Fig. 10

Commisura and Crura fornicis

Usual findings. Schematical topograms for Fig. 11
A to D   Transectional planes according to Fig. 11

Abbreviations
a   Commissura fornicis
(a)   as a, projection
b   Splenium corporis callosi
c   Corpus fornicis
d   Crus fornicis
e   Transitional area of Gyrus dentatus and Striae corporis callosi and of Gyrus cinguli
f   Striae of Gyrus cinguli before merging to a compact bundle of fibers

FIG. 10

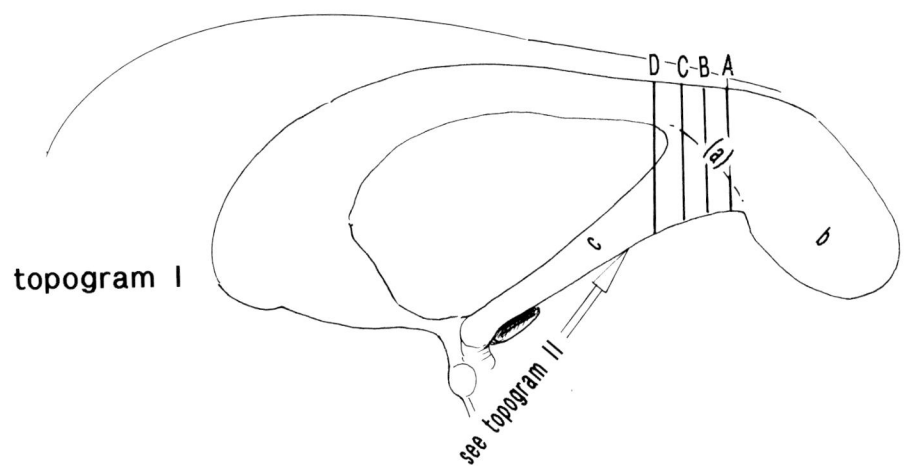

topogram I

see topogram II

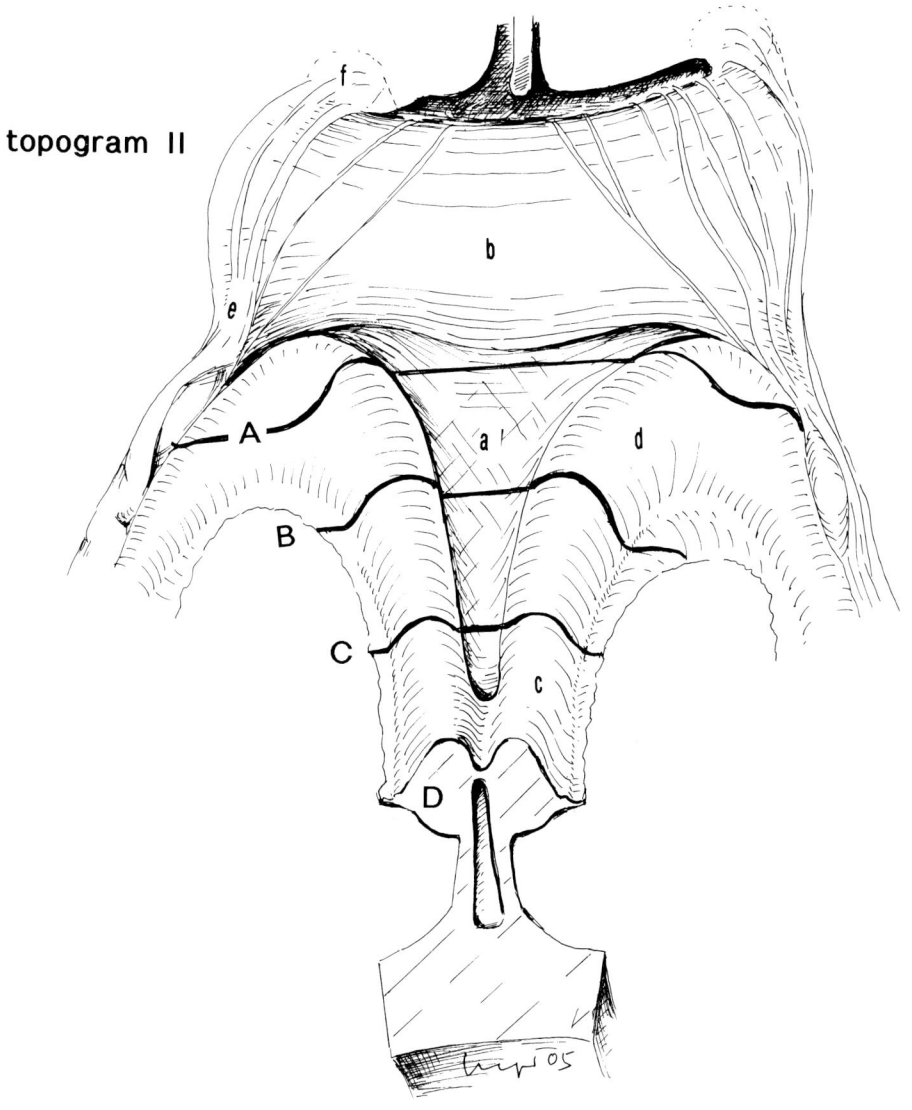

topogram II

Fig. 11

Continuation of Fig. 10

Coronal transections of Fornices, Fissura transversa and adjacent structures.
Sectional enlargements.

For topograms of transectional planes A to D see Fig. 10

Abbreviations
a, c, d as Fig. 10
b, e, f omitted
g   Corpus pineale
h   Habenula
i   Recessus suprapinealis
j   V. magna (Galeni)
k   V.basalis (Rosenthal)
l   V. cerebri int.
m   Velum interpositum
n   Fissura transversa
o   Atrium
p   Plexus chorioideus
q   Septum pellucidum
r   Cavum septi pellucidi

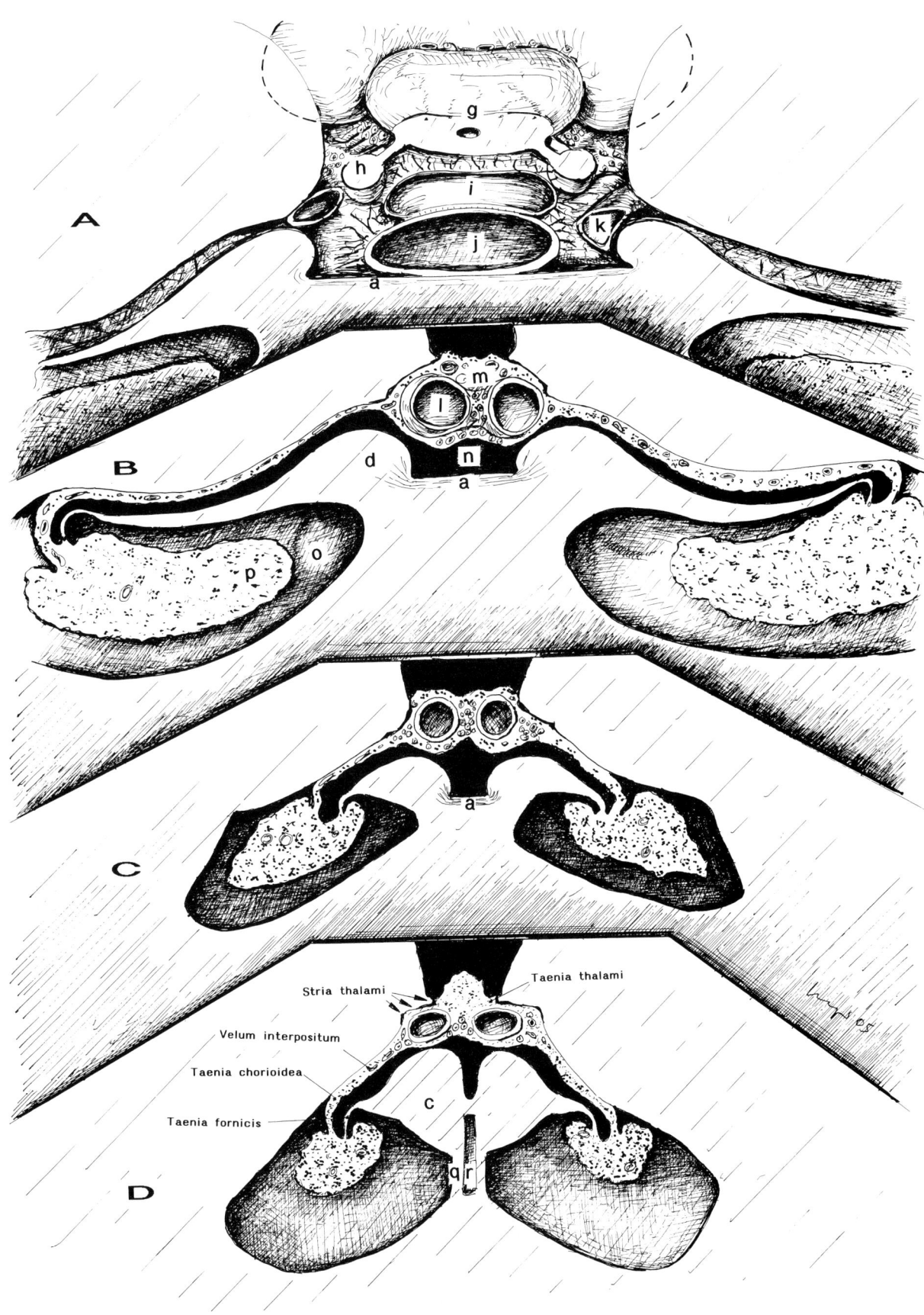

Stria thalami
Taenia thalami
Velum interpositum
Taenia chorioidea
Taenia fornicis

Fig. 12

Splenium corporis callosi and Tectum. Common findings
According to MRTs of normal individuals, simplified

Narrow distant measurements of Splenium and Tectum, especially Corpus pineale. At
surgery, the galenic vein may be loosened and lateralized

Black arrows: Relationships of Splenium and Colliculi supp.

FIG. 12

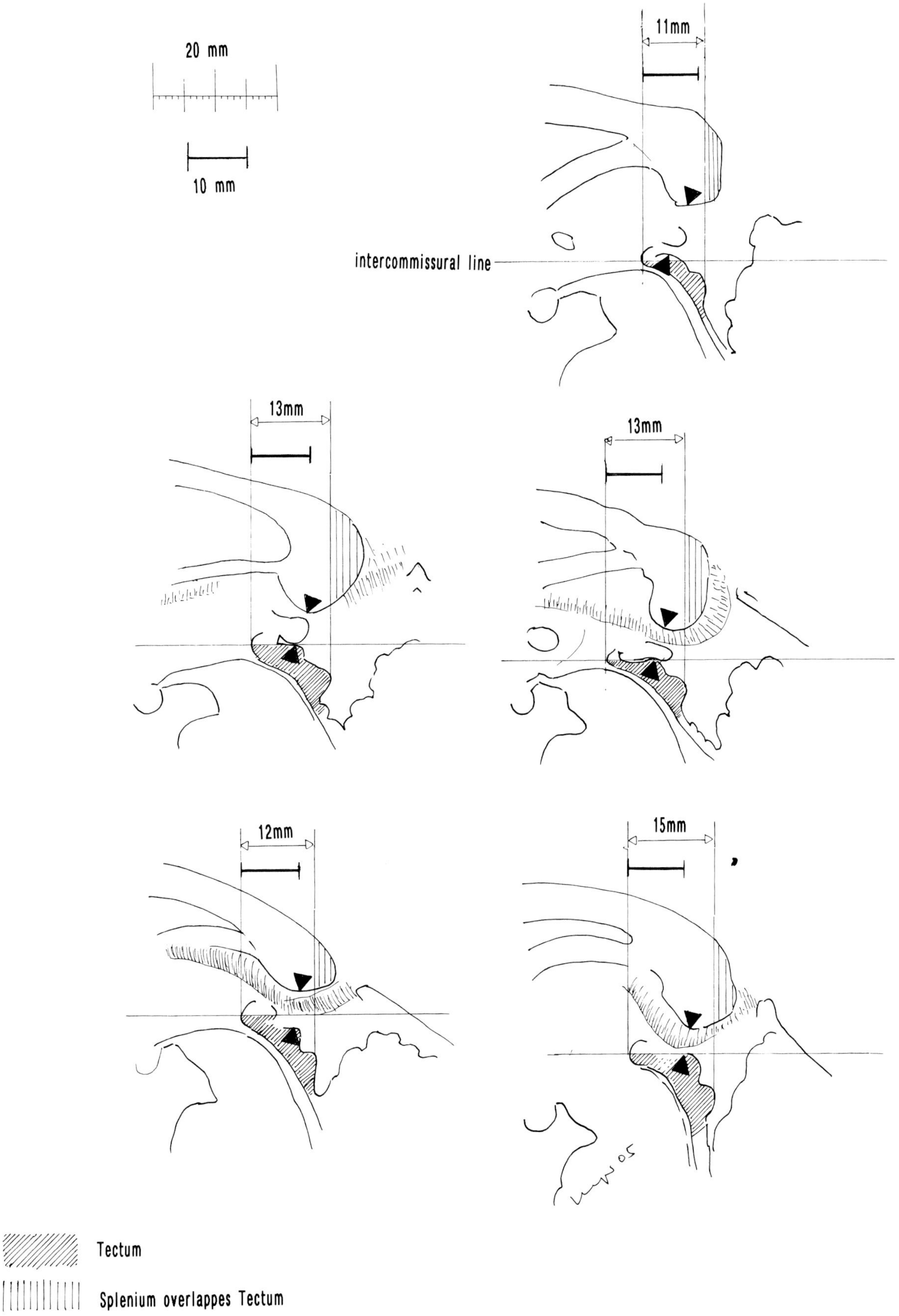

20 mm

10 mm

11mm

intercommissural line

13mm

13mm

12mm

15mm

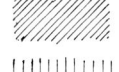

///// Tectum

||||||||| Splenium overlappes Tectum

Fig. 13

Tectum – Anatomical dissections

After removal of Arachnoidea and vessels

A   Tectum with Corpus pineale and its connections to Thalamus (Habenula)
B   Area of Habenula vulnerable. Here: Rupture of Commissura habenularum
      Fenestration after rupture between Corpus pineale and Tectum.
      After this, the 3rd ventricle is open with presentation of Commissura post.

Surgical aspects:
Injury to this area (and of the connection with Thalamus) must be taken in consideration

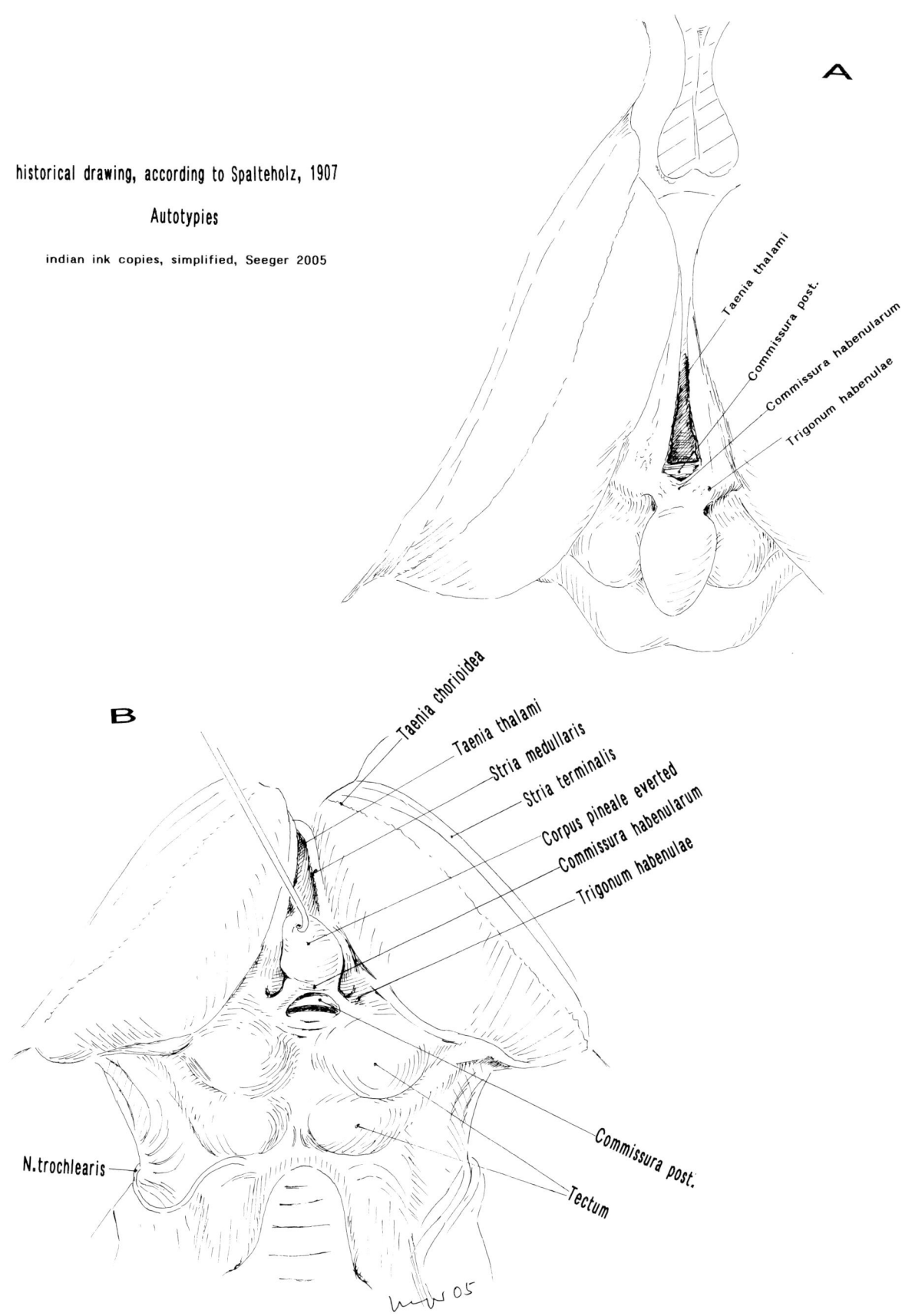

historical drawing, according to Spalteholz, 1907

Autotypies

indian ink copies, simplified, Seeger 2005

Fig. 14

Addendum for Fig. 13
Area of Habenula and surrounding structures of Aquaeductus

A   Simplified copy of a stained section of the brain, sectional enlarged (according to
Zuleger and Staubesand, 1977)
B   Sectional enlargement of A

Abbreviations
a   Velum interpositum, posterior limit area
b   Habenula
c   Nuclei habenulae
d   Commissura post.
e   Lemniscus medialis
f   Tractus segmentalis medialis
g   Fasciculus longitudinalis medialis
h   Nucleus ruber
i   Corpus geniculatum mediale
j   Corpus geniculatum laterale
k   Thalamus
l   Substantia nigra
m   Crus cerebri
n   Fossa interpeduncularis
o   N. oculomotorius
p   Pons
q   A. basilaris

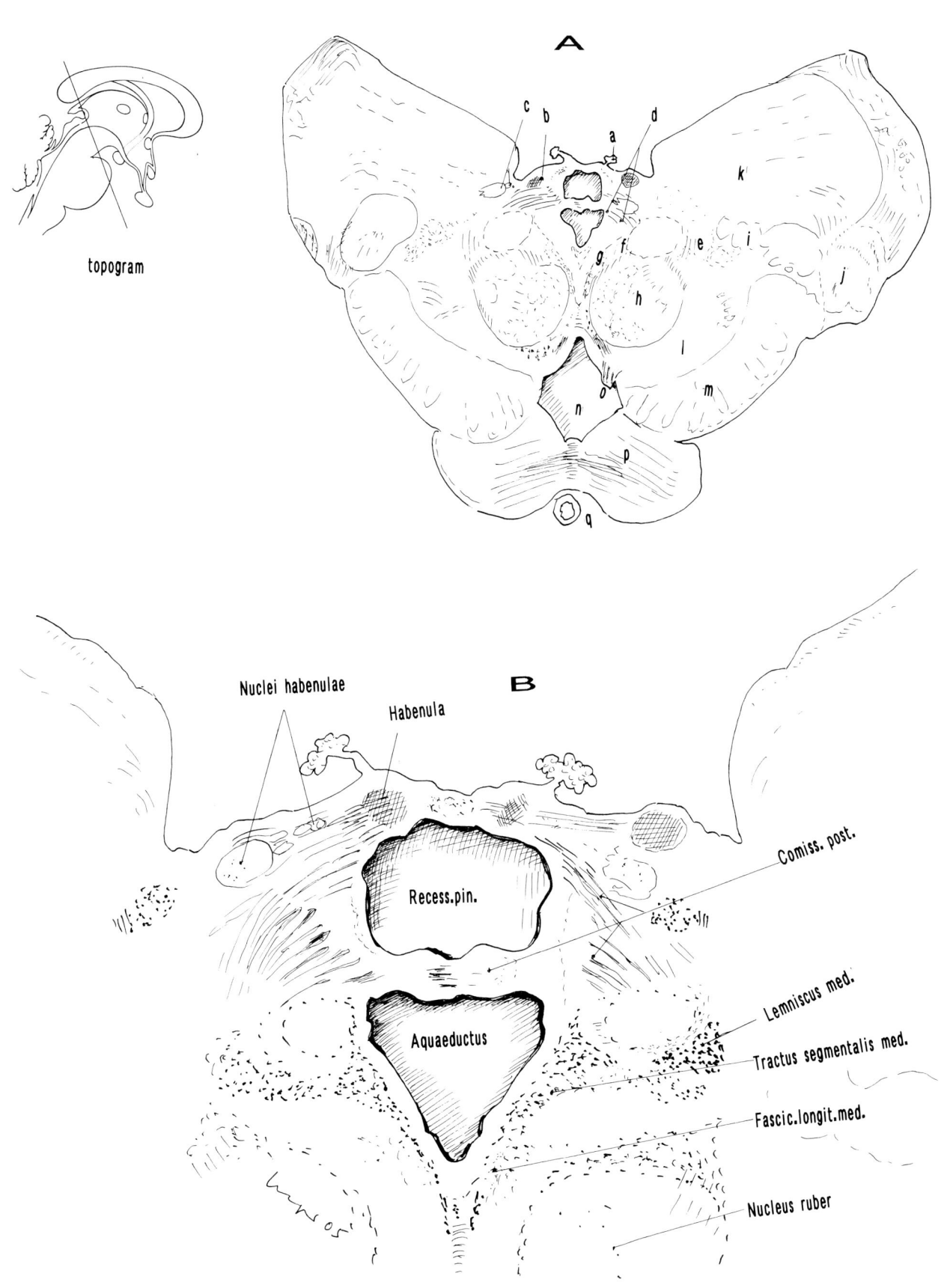

topogram

A

B

Nuclei habenulae

Habenula

Recess.pin.

Aquaeductus

Comiss. post.

Lemniscus med.

Tractus segmentalis med.

Fascic.longit.med.

Nucleus ruber

Fig. 15

Vessels of Cisterna ambiens, Cisterna tecti and of the bottom of Fissura transversa (Velum interpositum). Schematic anatomical drawings

A   Arteries and their relationships to veins
B   Veins, simplified

Abbreviations
a   V. magna (Galeni)
b   arachnoid membrane, enclosing Tentorium
c   V. supraculminalis
d   V. cerbellaris praecentralis
e   Vv. tecti

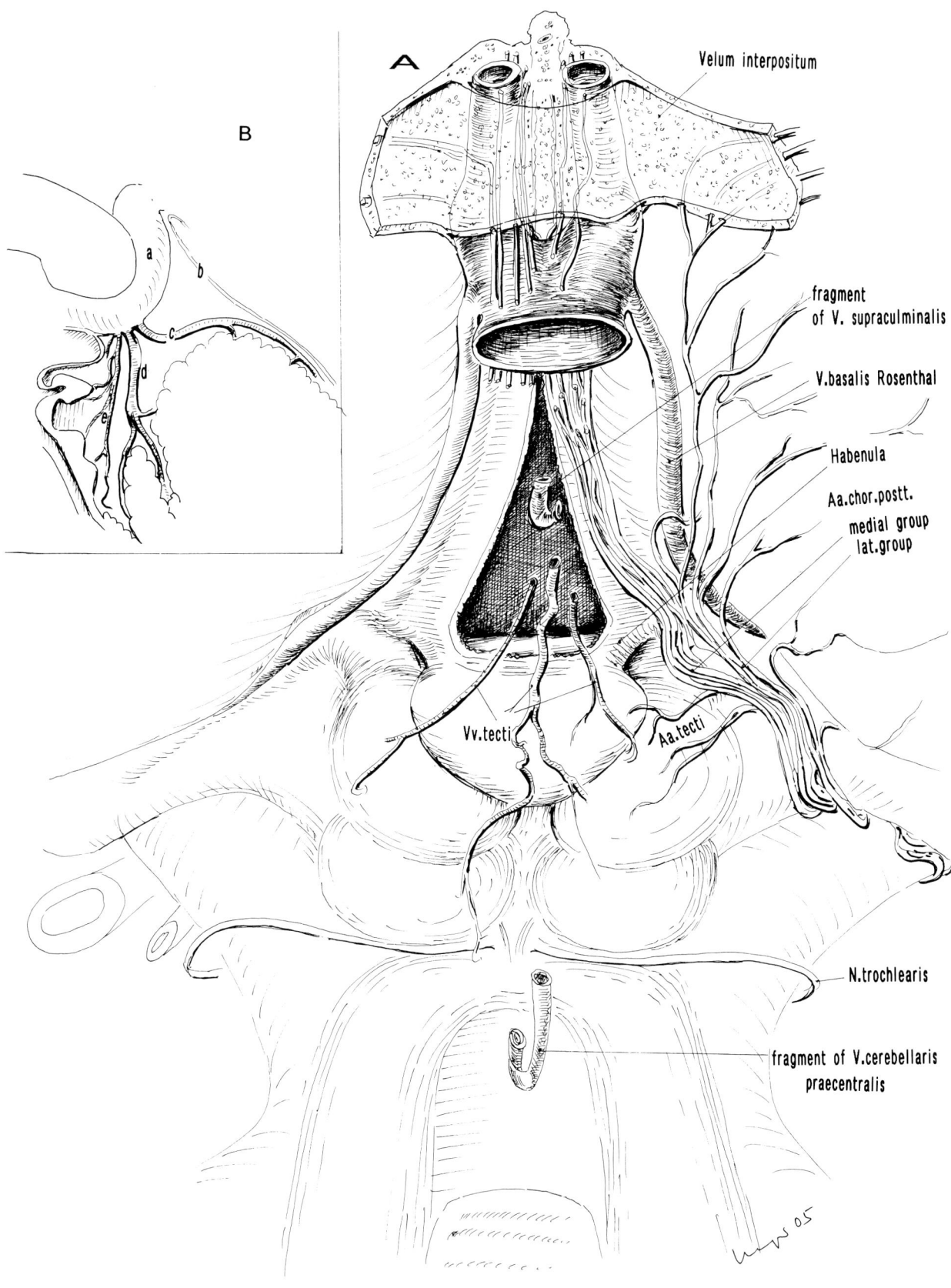

A

B

Velum interpositum

fragment
of V. supraculminalis

V.basalis Rosenthal

Habenula

Aa.chor.postt.
medial group
lat.group

Vv.tecti

Aa.tecti

N.trochlearis

fragment of V.cerebellaris
praecentralis

SURGICAL APPROACHES (Figs. 16 to 43)

Approaches crossing Lamina terminalis (Figs. 16 to 20)

Fig. 16

Principles of surgical approaches

– Subdural route between Falx and outer arachnoid layer (1st step)
– Incision of outer arachnoid layer along its fold at the margin of Falx. The subarachnoidal route crosses Sucus longitudinalis (Cisterna corporis callosi, 2nd step)
– Identification of Chiasma and Lamina terminalis between Areae subcallosae and
  between Gyri recti. The dorsal limit is Commissura ant. Median incision of Lamina
  terminalis and inspection of the 3rd ventricle (3rd step)

Abbreviations
a   Arachnoid fold along the margin of Falx
a'   as a, incised
b   Lamina terminalis
b'   as b, incised
c   Structures of the posterior area of the 3rd ventricle

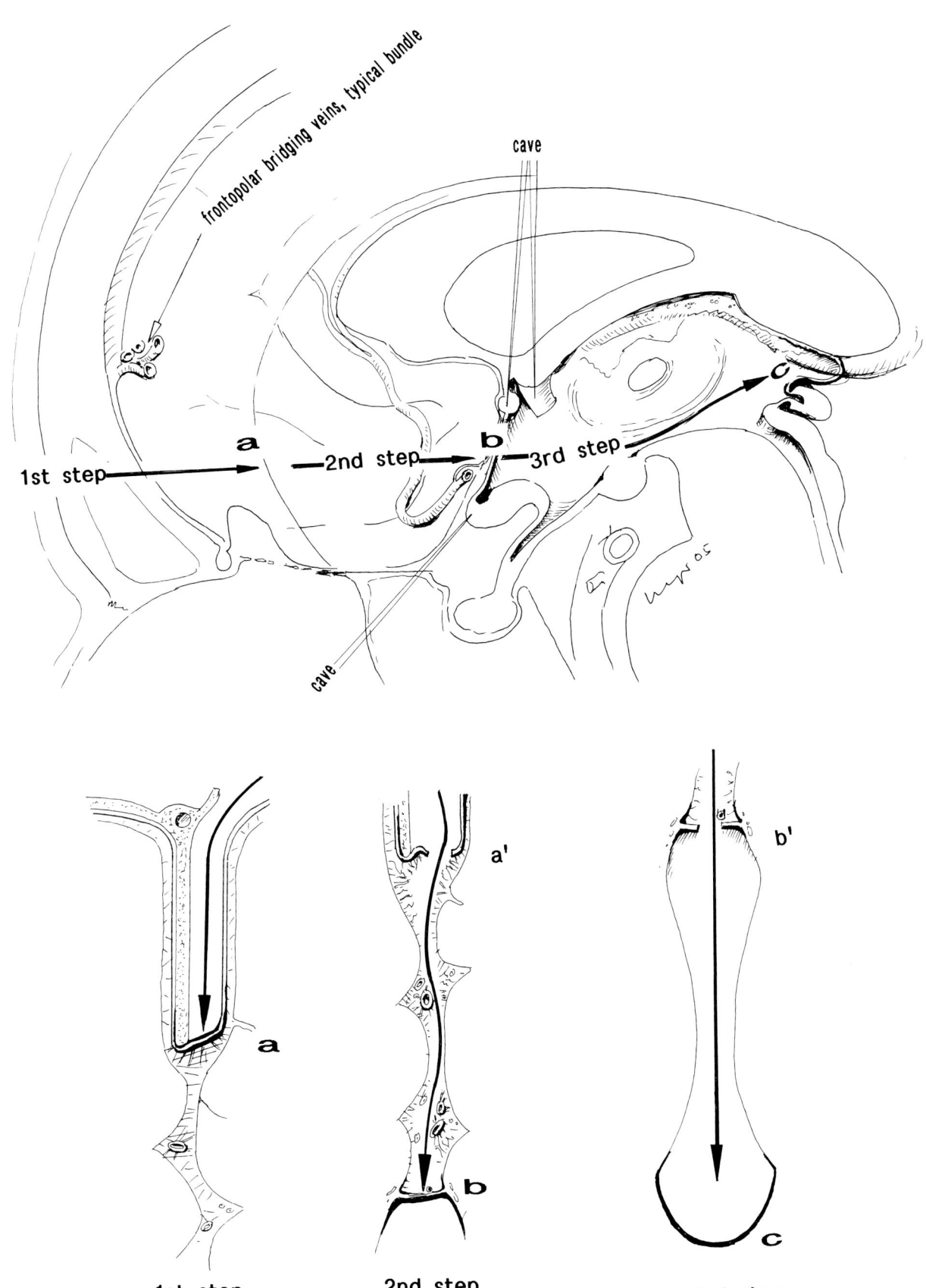

frontopolar bridging veins, typical bundle

cave

1st step

2nd step

3rd step

a

b

cave

1st step

2nd step

3rd step

a

a'

b

b'

c

Details (Figs. 17 and 18)

Fig. 17

Comparison of translaminar and transforaminal approaches

A Translaminar approaches
– Favorable:
Presentation of the posterior area of the 3rd ventricle
– Unfavorable:
Subdural approach along Falx sometimes may be obstructed by gaps of Falx.
It contains bifrontal subarachnoid adhesions

B Transforaminal approaches
– Favorable
The subdural route is less obstructed by adhesions
Short subarachnoid route
Variable approaches along a wide area of Falx may be used, if necessary
– Unfavorable
Surgical procedures in the posterior area of the 3rd ventricle are not possible.
This may be possible in the future. A combination with retroforaminal approaches is possible

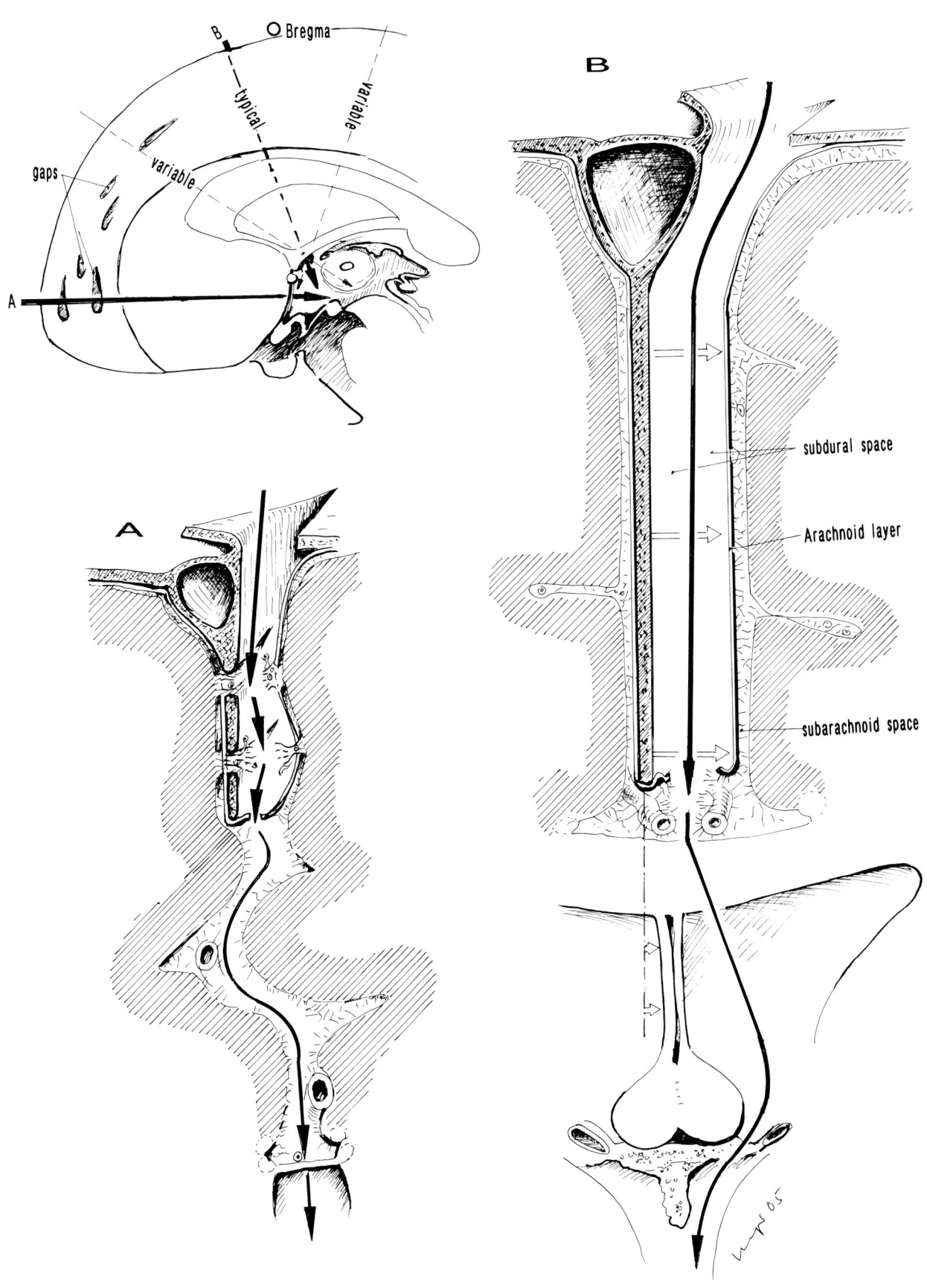

subdural space

Arachnoid layer

subarachnoid space

Fig. 18

Types of Lamina terminalis. Some surgical aspects

MRTs, simplified copies

FIG. 18

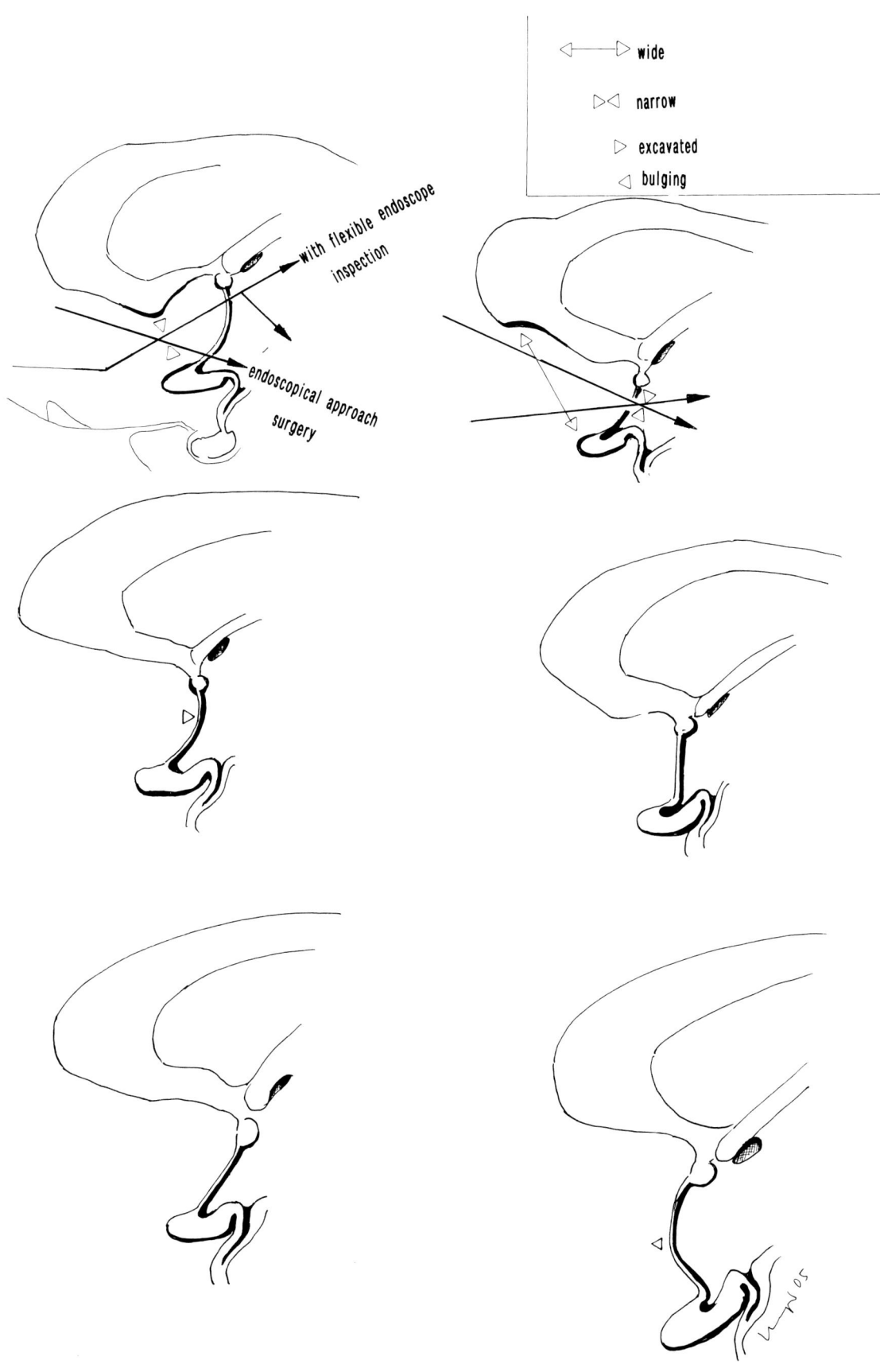

Intraventricular target areas (Figs. 19 and 20)

Fig. 19

Inspections by a flexible endoscope

A   Anatomical routes
B   Combination of multiple endoscopical topographies. Drawing according to a cadaver brain dissection

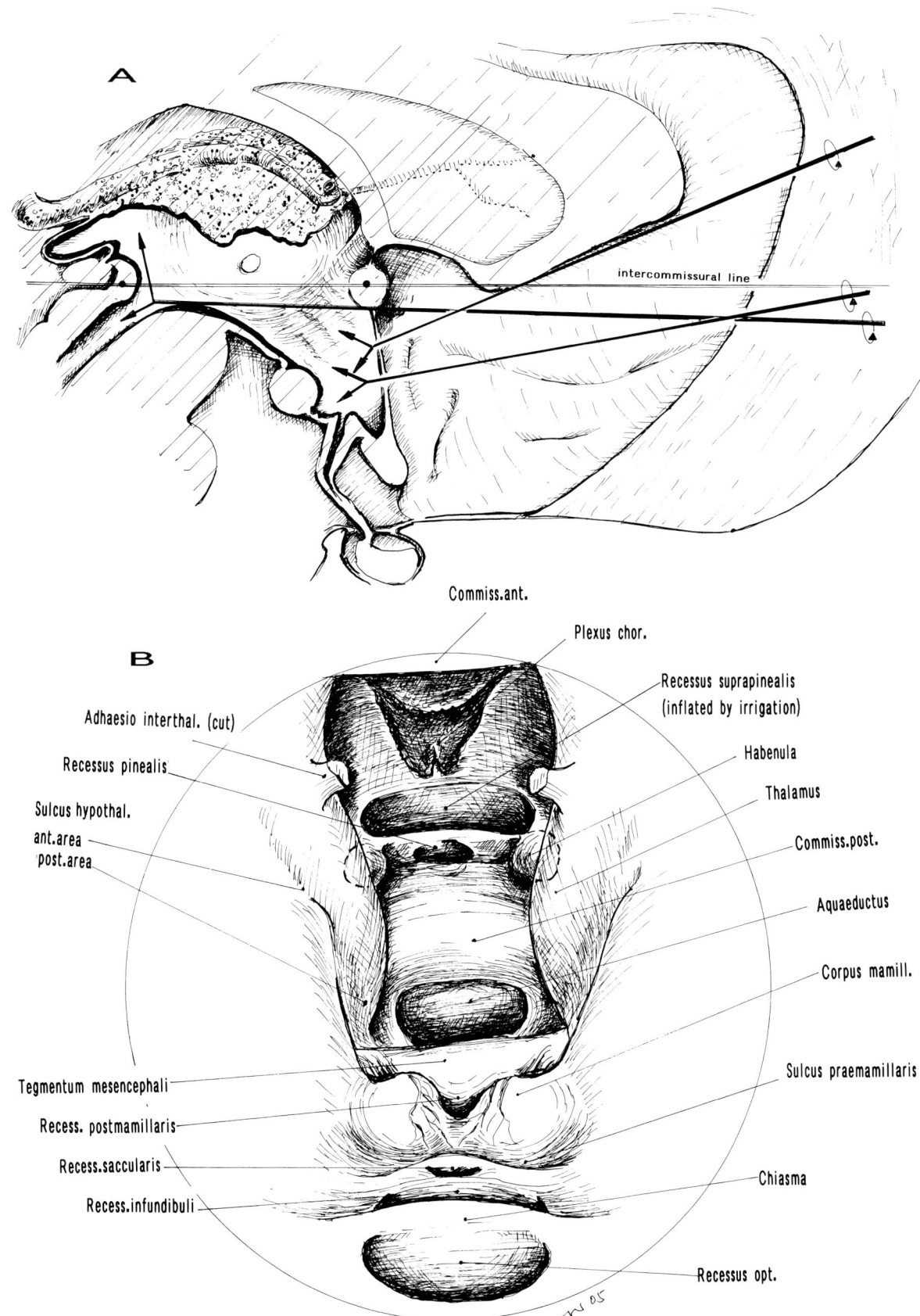

A

B

intercommissural line

Commiss.ant.

Plexus chor.

Recessus suprapinealis
(inflated by irrigation)

Adhaesio interthal. (cut)

Habenula

Recessus pinealis

Thalamus

Sulcus hypothal.

Commiss.post.

ant.area
post.area

Aquaeductus

Corpus mamill.

Tegmentum mesencephali

Sulcus praemamillaris

Recess. postmamillaris

Recess.saccularis

Chiasma

Recess.infundibuli

Recessus opt.

Fig. 20

Microsurgical topography or endoscopical topography using a non-flexible endoscope.
Drawing according to a cadaver brain dissection

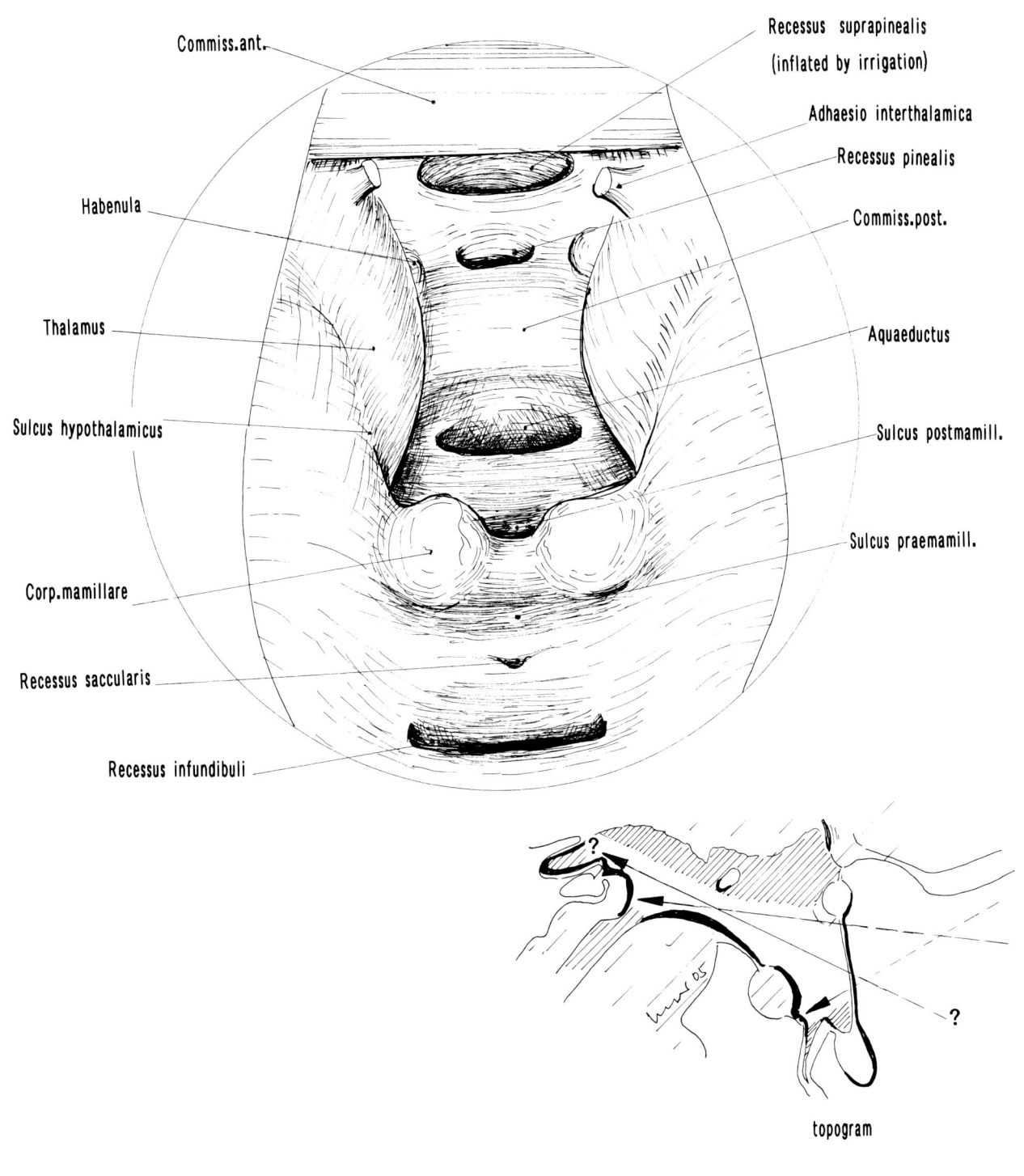

Commiss.ant.

Recessus suprapinealis
(inflated by irrigation)

Adhaesio interthalamica

Recessus pinealis

Commiss.post.

Habenula

Thalamus

Aquaeductus

Sulcus hypothalamicus

Sulcus postmamill.

Sulcus praemamill.

Corp.mamillare

Recessus saccularis

Recessus infundibuli

topogram

not to be presented

Approaches transcrossing Foramen interventriculare (Monroi) (Figs. 21 to 30)

Fig. 21

Principles of surgical approaches

– Incision of the skin, of Galea and Periosteum.
  Trepanation. Incision of Dura. Subdural route along Falx.
  Presention of the fold of arachnoid layer along the margin of Falx (1st step)
– Incision of the fold of arachnoid layer along the margin of Falx.
  Crossing of the small segment of Cisterna corporis callosi
  Incision of Corpus callosum. Crossing of the lateral ventricle
  Presentation of Foramen interventriculare (2nd step)
– Crossing Foramen interventriculare
  Presentation of the anterior area of the 3rd ventricle (3rd step)

Abbreviation
a   Arachnoid fold at the margin of Falx, enlarged before incision
a'   as a, after incision
b   Foramen interventriculare
b'   as b, after crossing
c   floor of the 3rd ventricle

FIG. 21

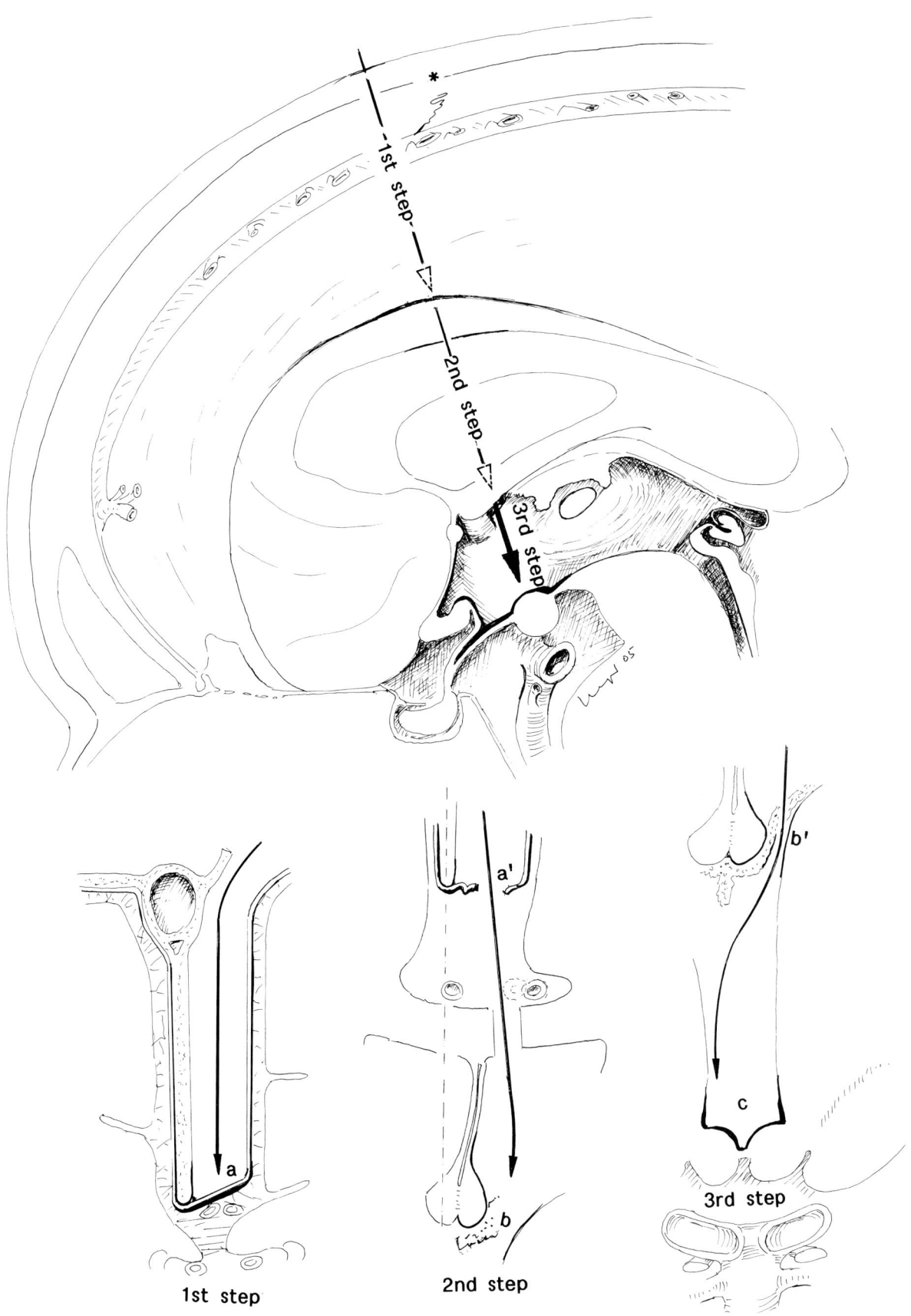

1st step

2nd step

3rd step

Details (Figs. 22 to 28)

Fig. 22

Defining of Foramen interventriculare (Monroi) by MRT, principles

A   *1* Usual route
      2 If the presentation of the interventricular foramen by MRT is unclear (overlapped by a hyperlastic plexus or flattening of its margin by a space-occupying lesion, e.g.), its definition may be inexact. Now it is useful to define Bregma and Corpora mamillaria. The interventricular foramen is located at a straight connection line between Bregma and Corpora mamillaria.

B   Relationships of the interventricular foramen to Commissura ant. and to the intercommissural line:
      The distance measurements between the interventricular foramen and of the intercommissural line vary from 3 to 5 mm

These measurements are sufficient for microsurgery and endoscopy, but not sufficient for blind stereotactic punctures.

FIG. 22

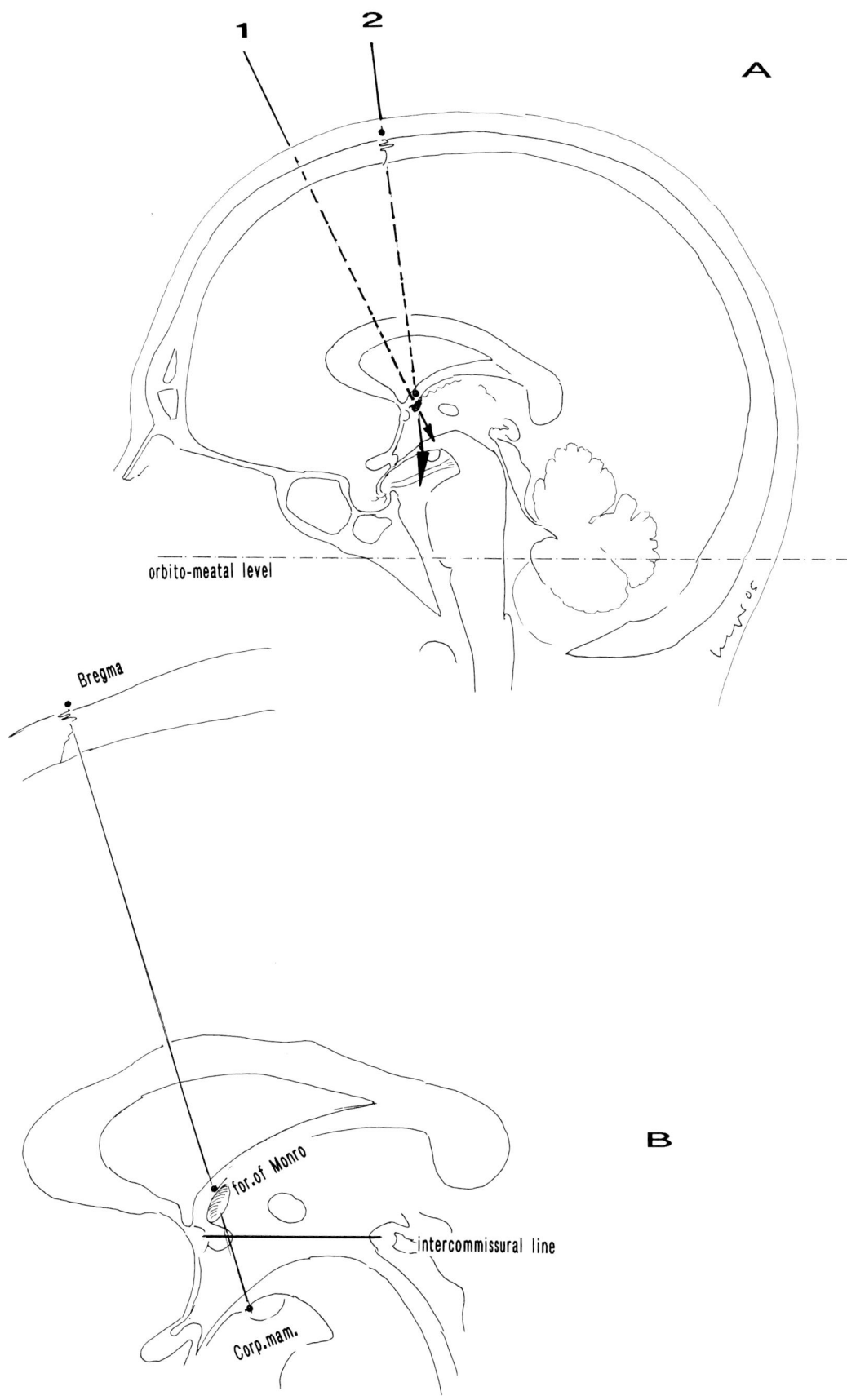

A

orbito-meatal level

Bregma

for.of Monro

intercommissural line

Corp.mam.

B

Fig. 23

Variable dorsal midline approaches

FIG. 23

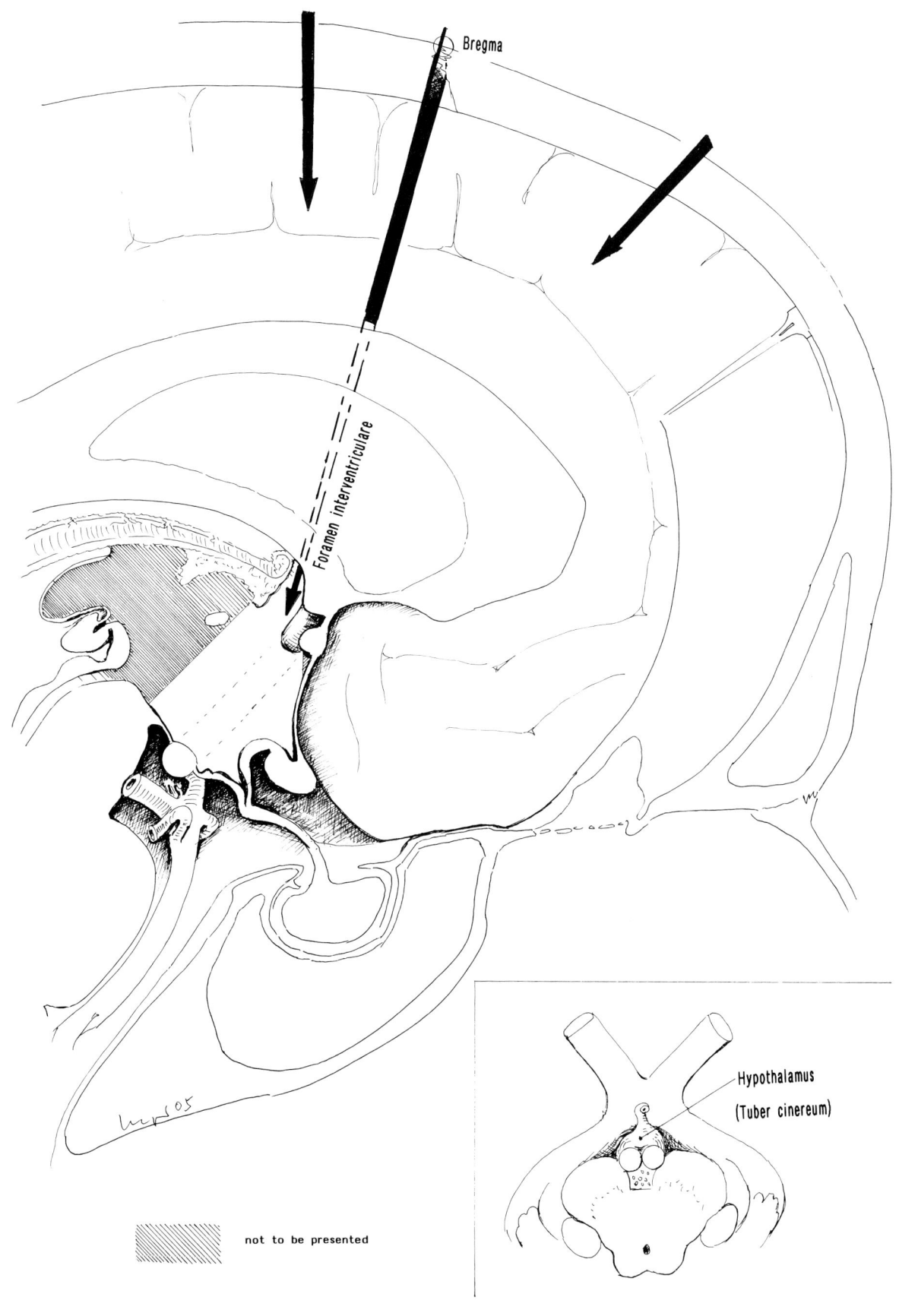

Bregma

Foramen interventriculare

Hypothalamus
(Tuber cinereum)

not to be presented

Fig. 24

Avoiding bridging veins

The variable bridging veins may complicate the dorsal midline approaches close to the sinus
Imaging strategies help to find out the favorable routes. The bridging veins should be preserved, as well as possible. Careful surgical procedures are possible between the veins. The location of the target areas of the 3rd ventricle must be taken in consideration.
Arrows: surgical approaches.

A Bregma may be used as a landmark. It can be defined by palpation (see B), by CT or MRT. After this, it may be marked by a silicon tube, e.g.. In a fMRT the relationship of veins and Bregma can be identified
B Palpation and definition of Bregma. In many individuals, this method is sufficient
C Widening of the target areas using variable routes

FIG. 24

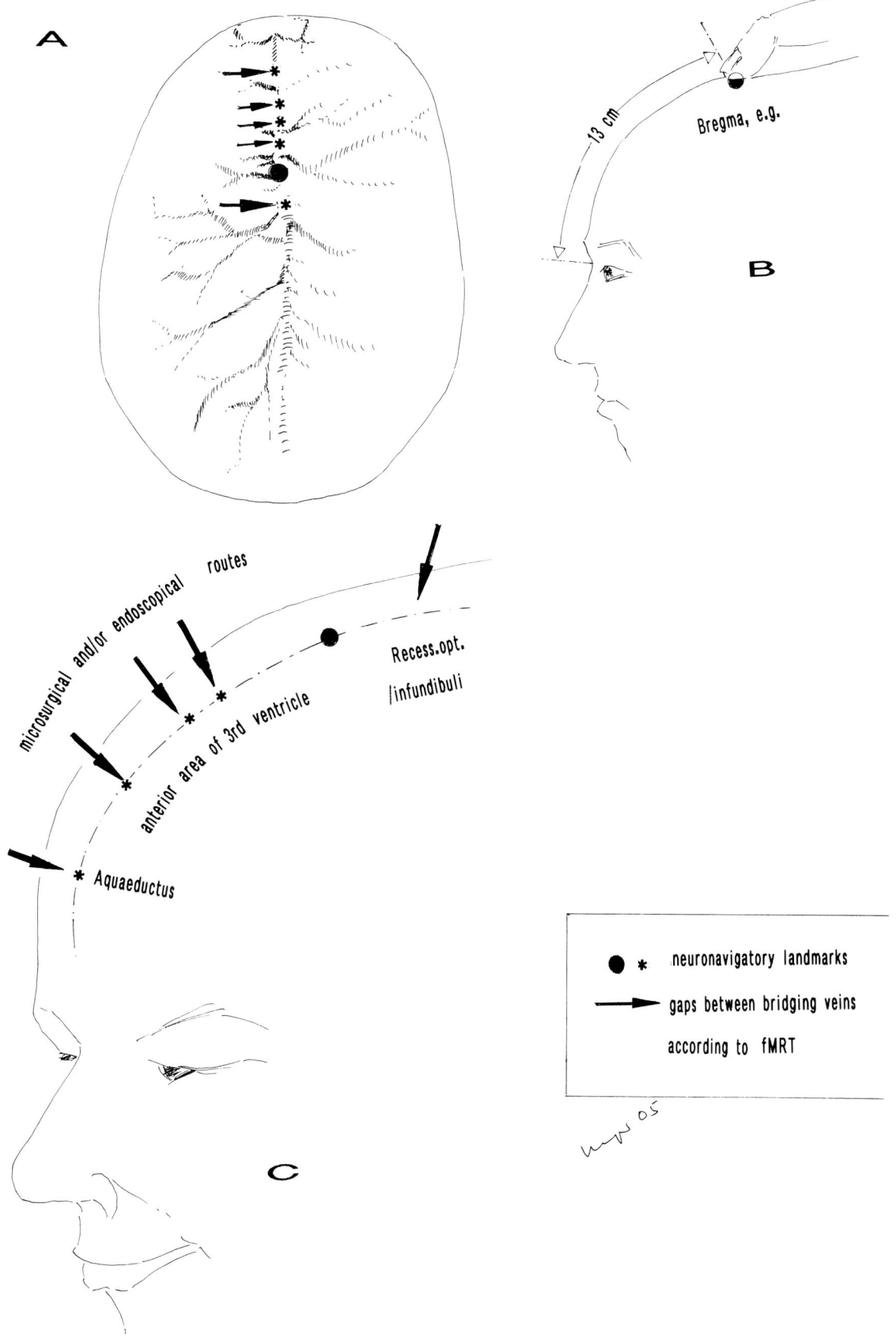

A

B

Bregma, e.g.

13 cm

microsurgical and/or endoscopical routes

anterior area of 3rd ventricle

Recess.opt. /infundibuli

* Aquaeductus

C

● * neuronavigatory landmarks

→ gaps between bridging veins according to fMRT

Fig. 25

Incision of Corpus callosum

A   Cisterna corporis callosi and surrounding structures
A'   Addendum für A
B   Surgical route. Preservation of allocortical structures, as good as possible. Fine fibers (see A) useful fo landmarks
    Avoiding of opening of the contralateral ventricle
C   After incision of Corpus callosum in a sagittal direction, its inner layer (Ependyma) should be split in a transversal direction for preservation of veins

Abbreviations
a   allocortical stria of Gyrus cinguli
b   Striae corporis callosi latt.
c   Striae corporis callosi medd.
d   allocortical bundles of fibers
e   neocortical bundles (fibers of Corpus callosum alternating with d)
f   Gyrus cinguli
g   Corpus callosum
h   Ventriculus lat.
i   Septum pellucidum
j   Foramen interventriculare Monroi

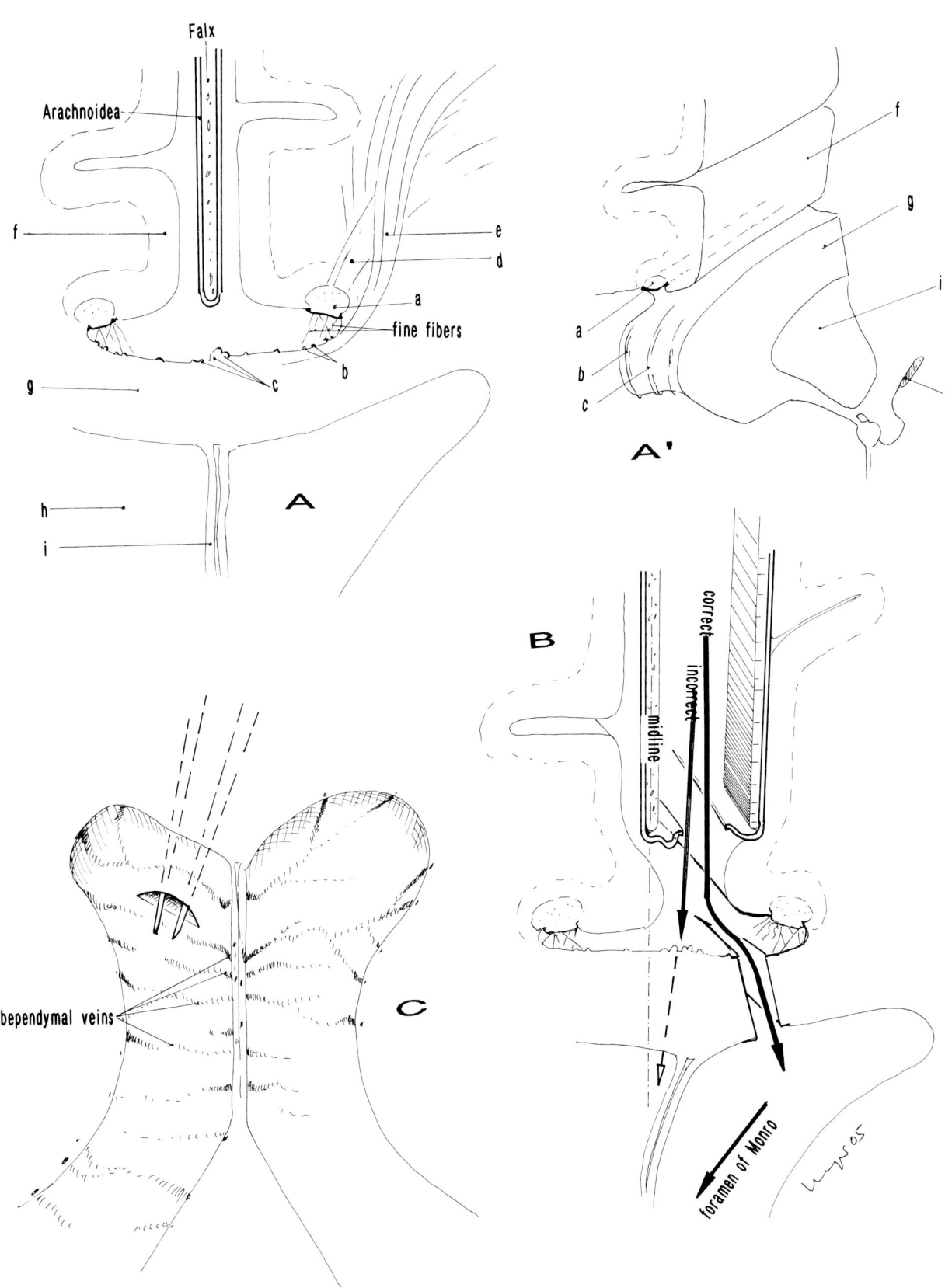

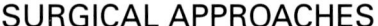

Fig. 26

Anatomical drawings for understanding preoperative MRTs

Comparison of the intraventricular structures and its relationships to adjacent structures

FIG. 26

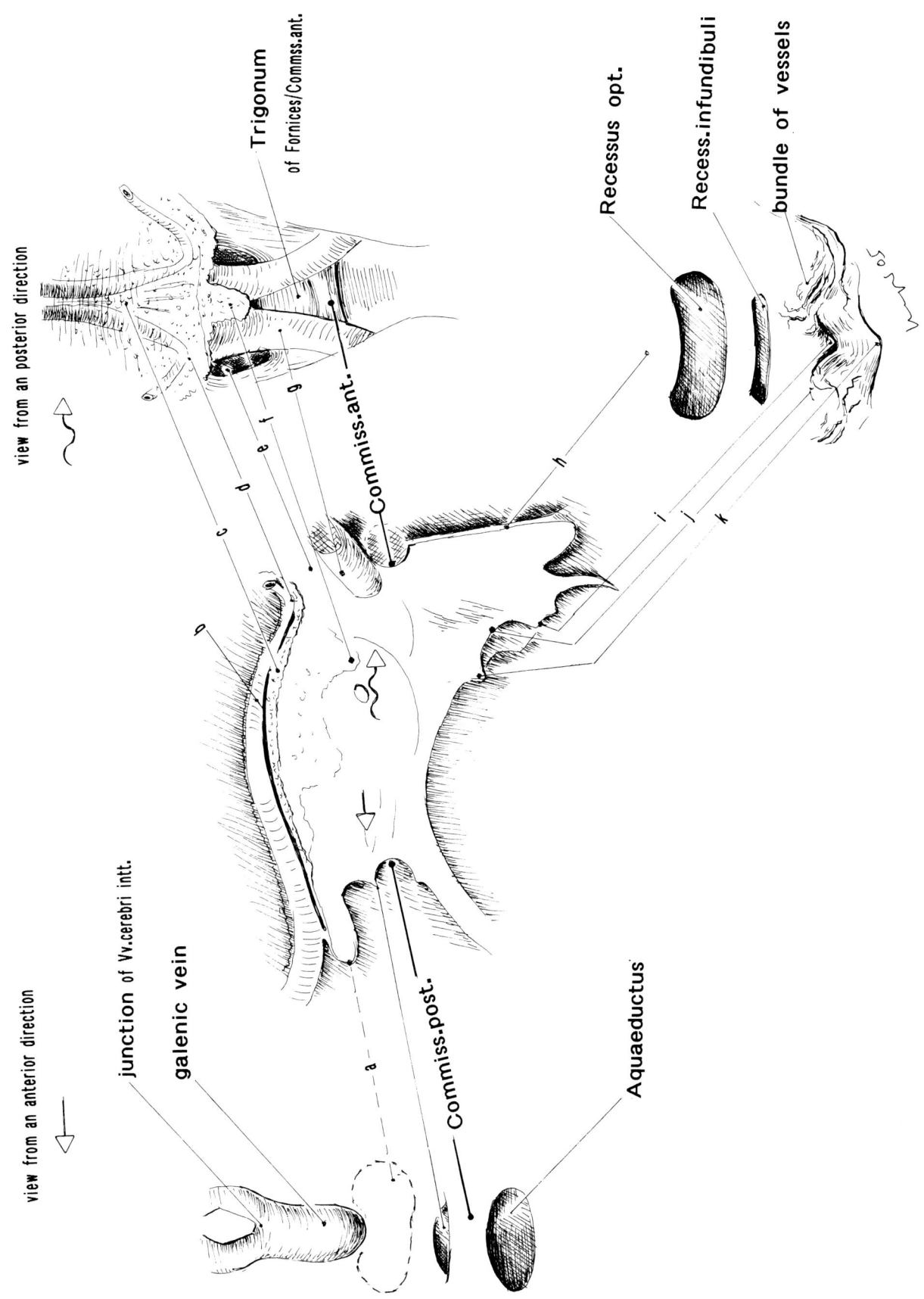

view from an posterior direction

Trigonum
of Fornices/Commiss.ant.

Commiss.ant.

Recessus opt.

Recess.infundibuli

bundle of vessels

junction of Vv.cerebri intt.

galenic vein

view from an anterior direction

Commiss.post.

Aquaeductus

Fig. 27

Continuation of Fig. 26
Adjacent structures

– Different views according to endoscopical approaches
– Drawing of structures surrounding the 3rd ventricle
– Periventricular details as seen in microsurgical and/or endoscopical approaches before reaching the 3rd ventricle

Abbreviations *a* to *l* according to Fig. 26

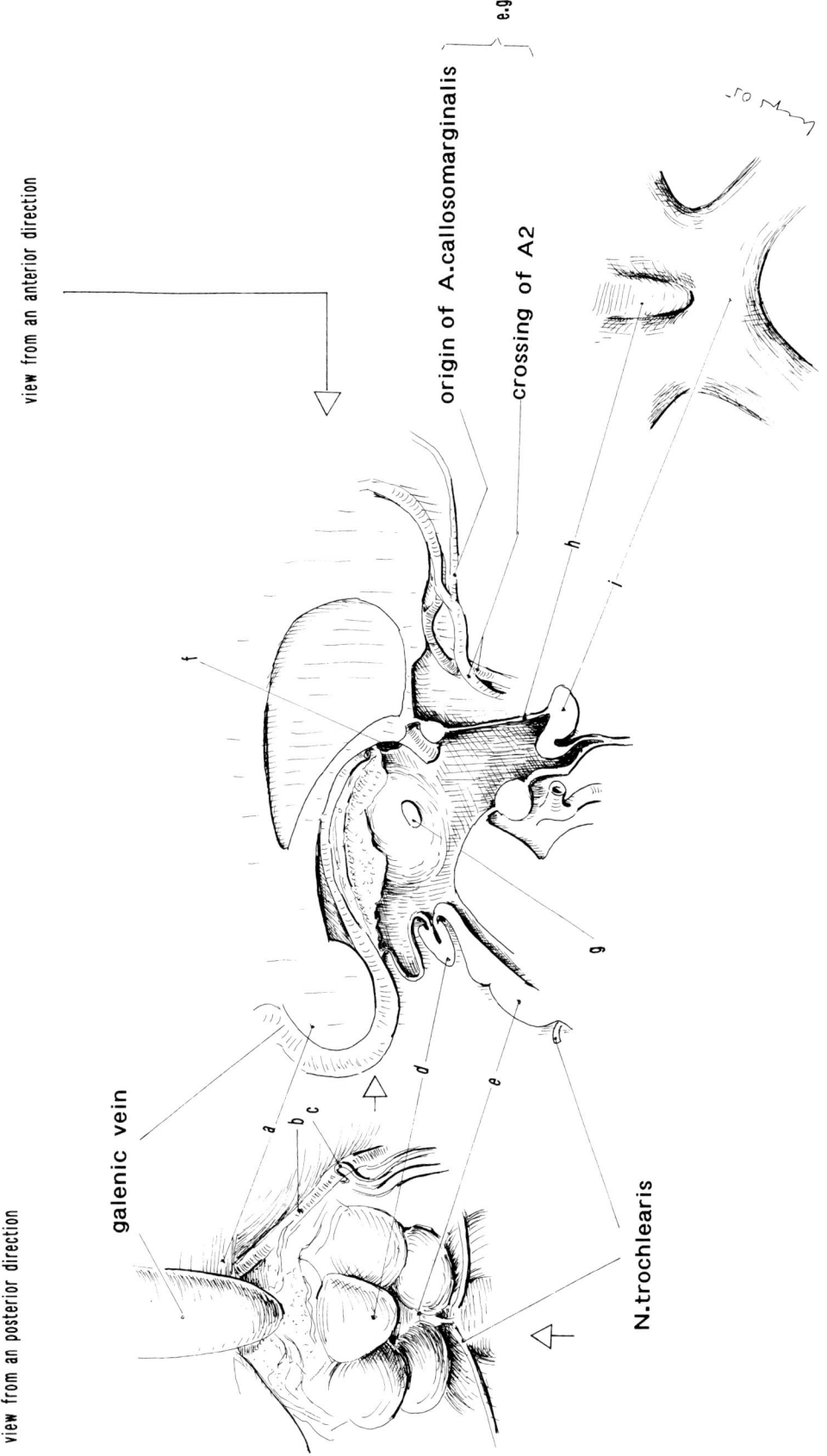

view from an anterior direction

view from an posterior direction

galenic vein

N.trochlearis

origin of A.callosomarginalis

crossing of A2

e.g.

Fig. 28

Incision of Corpus callosum. Surgical topography

A and **A'**   One or more branches of A. pericallosa cross the midline and feed areas of
                 the contralateral hemispehre. These are normal findings. An interruption of
                 it may be followed by a contralateral encephalomalazia (Marino 1976)

B   Microsurgical topography. Presentation of the anterior area of Corpus cal-
                 losum, beginning at Genu corporis callosi

FIG. 28

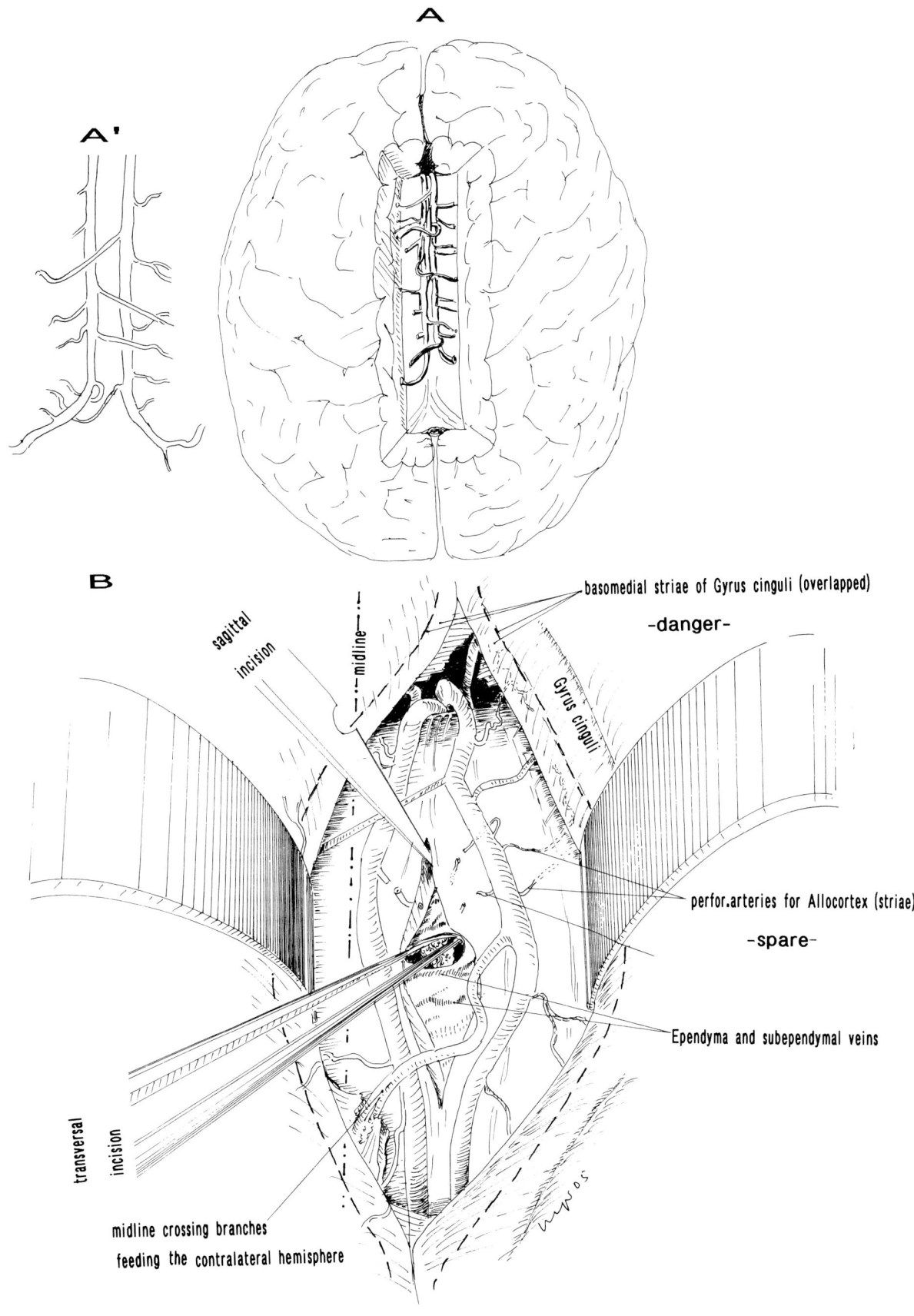

A

A'

B

basomedial striae of Gyrus cinguli (overlapped)

-danger-

sagittal incision

midline

Gyrus cinguli

perfor.arteries for Allocortex (striae)

-spare-

Ependyma and subependymal veins

transversal incision

midline crossing branches
feeding the contralateral hemisphere

Fig. 29

Surgical topography of the third ventricle crossing Foramen interventriculare (Monroi)

The foramen is widened by a space occupying lesion, which was eliminated
Topogram (anatomical sketch)

– Black shaped: Target areas at a straight approach
– Black arrow: Main surgical approach
– Light arrows: Variants of midline routes

Abbreviations
a   Commissura ant.
b   Fornix, Pars tecta (projection)
c   Chiasma, posterior from Recessus opt.
d   Recessus infundibuli
e   Recessus saccularis
f   Sulcus praemamillaris
g   Corpora mamillaria
h   Sulcus hypothalamicus
i   Thalamus

FIG. 29

topogram

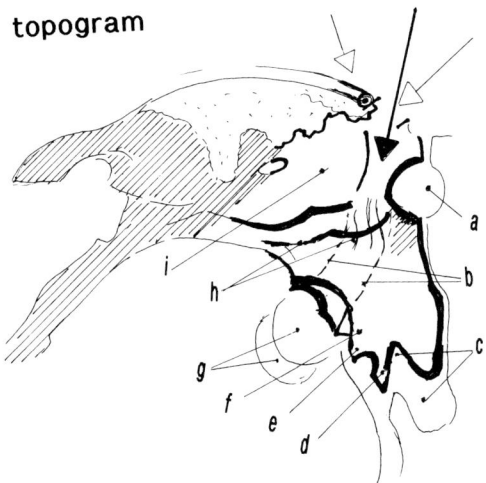

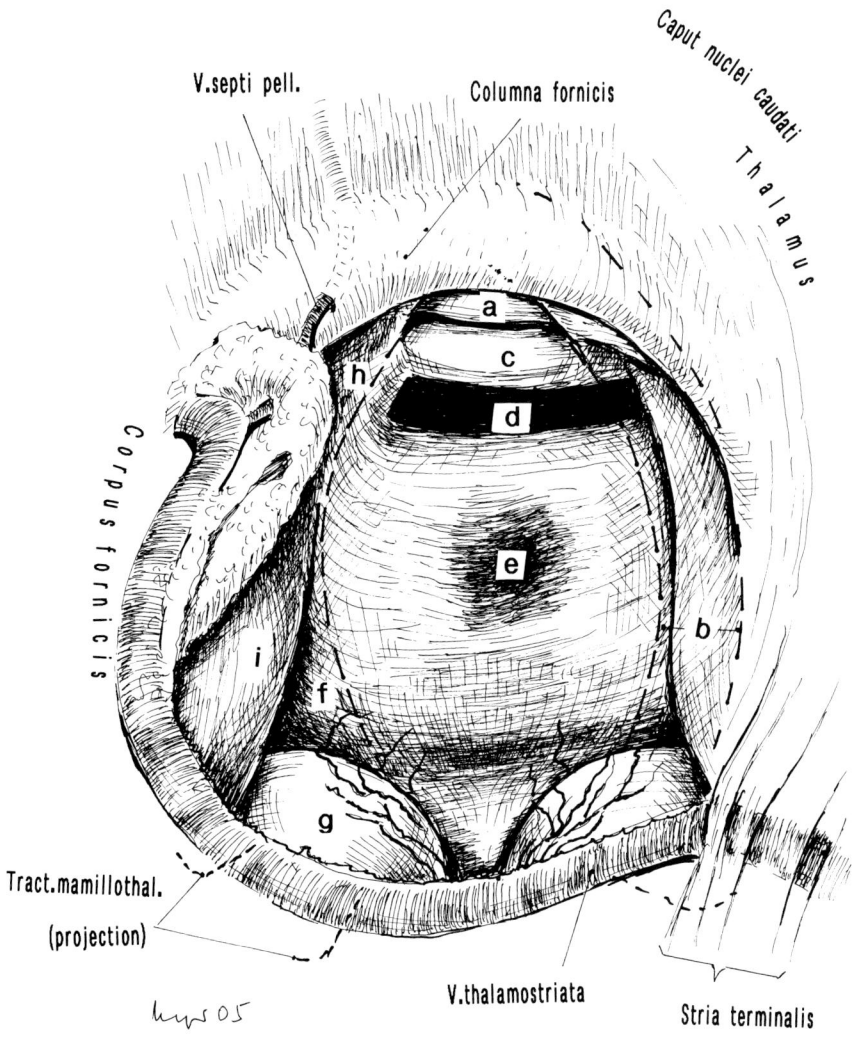

Fig. 30

Retroforaminal widening of a narrow variant of Foramen interventriculare (Monroi)

A   Connection of a thickened medial septal vein with V. thalamostriata
Fusion of Thalamus and Corpus fornicis combined with a deficit of Taenia chorioidea et fornicis in this area*

B   Transforaminal surgical approach widened to a retroforaminal approach
An alternative approach may be recommended: The retroforaminal interfornical
approach of Apuzzo et al, 1982

Abbreviations
a   Recessus infundibuli
b   Corpus mamillare
c   Columna fornicis
c'   as *c*, contralateral side
d   Thalamus
d'   Pars affixa thalami, after transection of its connection with Fornix
e   Chiasma
f   as *a*

———————

* Seeger 1988 pp 248 ff

FIG. 30

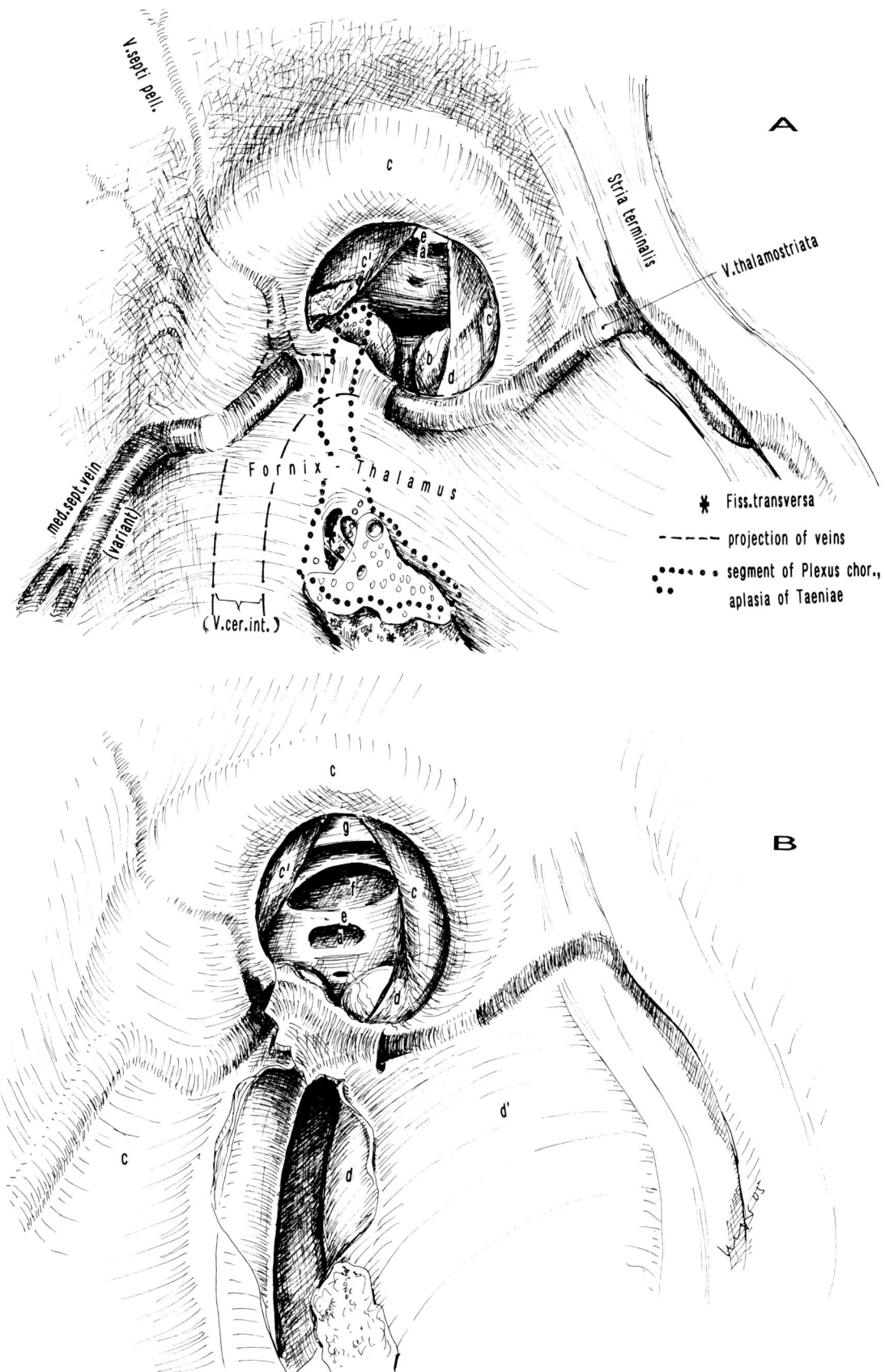

A

V.septi pell.

c

e
a
c'
c'
b d
c

Stria terminalis

V.thalamostriata

med.sept.vein
(variant)

Fornix - Thalamus

(V.cer.int.)

✳ Fiss.transversa

- - - - - projection of veins

• • • • • • segment of Plexus chor.,
aplasia of Taeniae

B

c

g
c'
f
c
e
d

c

d

d'

Approaches crossing Fissura transversa – retroforaminal approaches –
(Figs. 31 to 36)

Fig. 31

Principles of surgical approaches

A – 2 examples of the variable approaches
Midline approaches as in transforaminal approaches until the lateral ventricle is opened
– Further surgical steps see B and C

B Route for the anterior segment of the 3rd ventricle

C Route for the posterior segment of the 3rd ventricle

Abbreviations
a typical bridging vein(s)
b Sin. sagitt. inf.
c V. cerebri int.
d Fissura transversa cerebri
e foramen of Monroi
f Fornix, Pars tecta
(f) as f, projection
g Corpus mamillare
(g) as g, projection
h Recessus infundibuli
i Commissura post.
j Corpus pineale and its recessus
k Recessus suprapinealis
l Sulcus hypothalamicus, here: flattened
m Aquaeductus
n Chiasma
o Recessus opt.

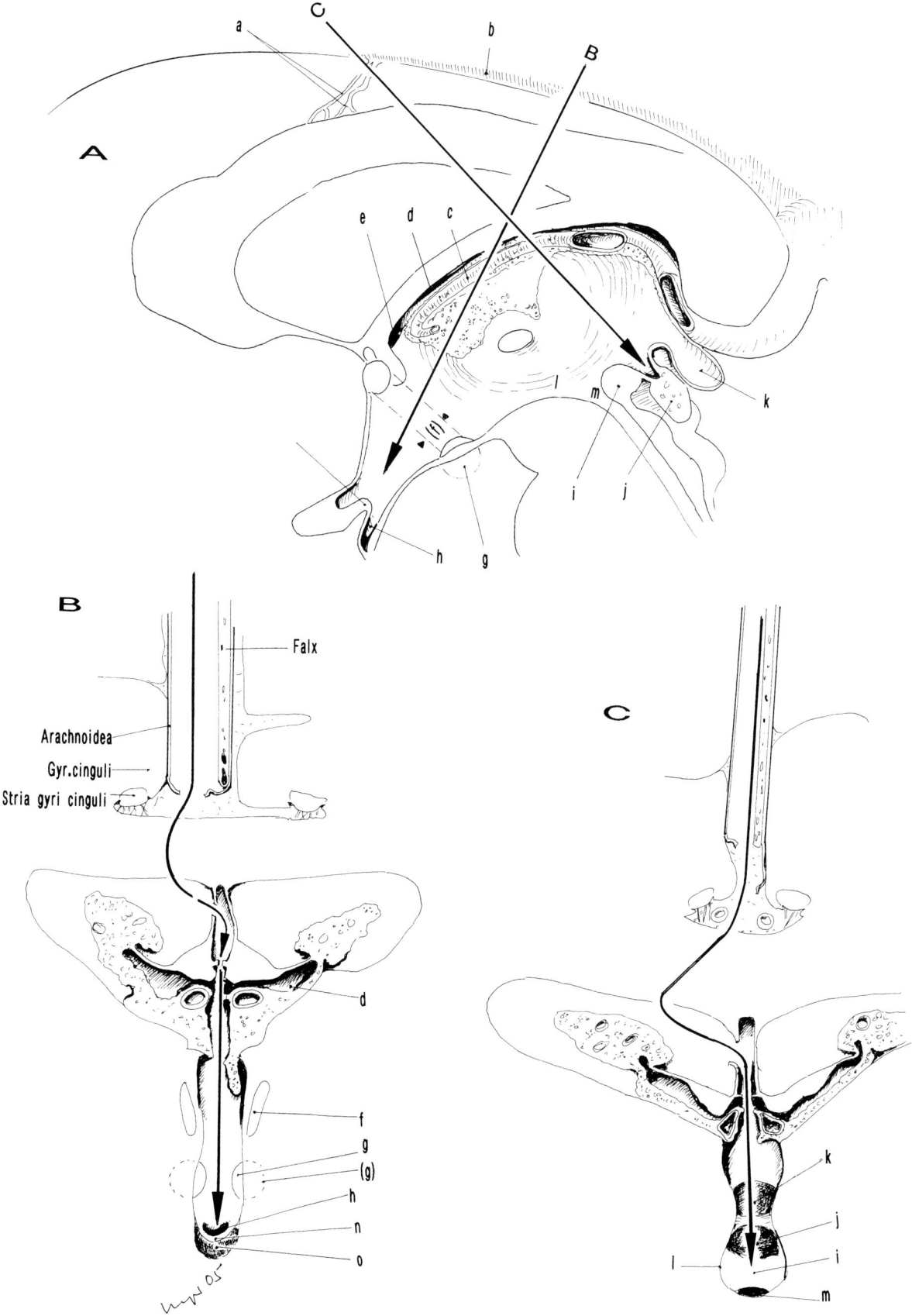

A

B

Falx

Arachnoidea

Gyr.cinguli

Stria gyri cinguli

C

Fig. 32

Avoiding bridging veins

The principles of these surgical procedures are the same as for transforaminal approaches (see Fig. 24):

A and **B** Bregma may be used as a landmark
C   Widening of the target areas using variable routes

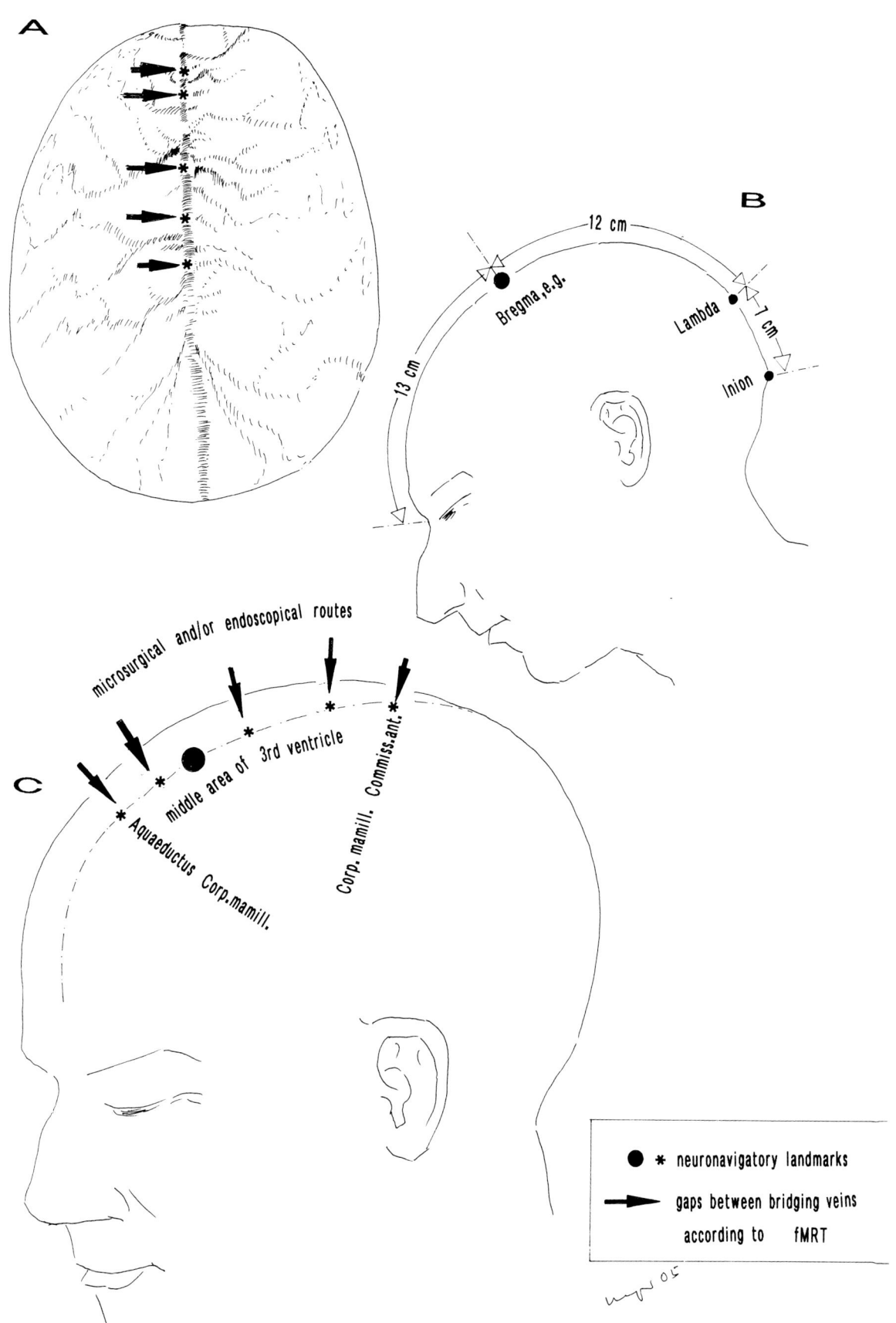

A

B

12 cm

13 cm

Bregma, e.g.

Lambda

7 cm

Inion

C

microsurgical and/or endoscopical routes

middle area of 3rd ventricle

Aquaeductus Corp.mamill.

Corp. mamill. Commiss.ant.

● * neuronavigatory landmarks

➡ gaps between bridging veins

according to fMRT

Fig. 33

Avoiding damage of a prefixed Fornix

This common variant is defined by MRT

There are two types of surgical approaches, depending on the target areas:
– Approaches for the anterior target areas, see A to C
– Approaches for the posterior target areas, see Fig. 34

A Routes to the anterior target areas of the 3rd ventricle

B Wide variant of the posterior end of Cavum septi pellucidi. This segment is often a little widened. This is favorable for the interfornical splitting

C Small variant of the posterior end of Cavum septi pellucidi

Abbreviations
a Corpus callosum
b Septum pellucidum
c Columna fornicis
d Fissura transversa cerebri
e V. cerebri int.
f V. magna (Galeni)
g Velum interpositum and Plexus chor. of the 3rd ventricle
h Thalamus, ventricular surface
i Corpus mamillare
n stria of Gyrus cinguli (see Fig. 34)

FIG. 33

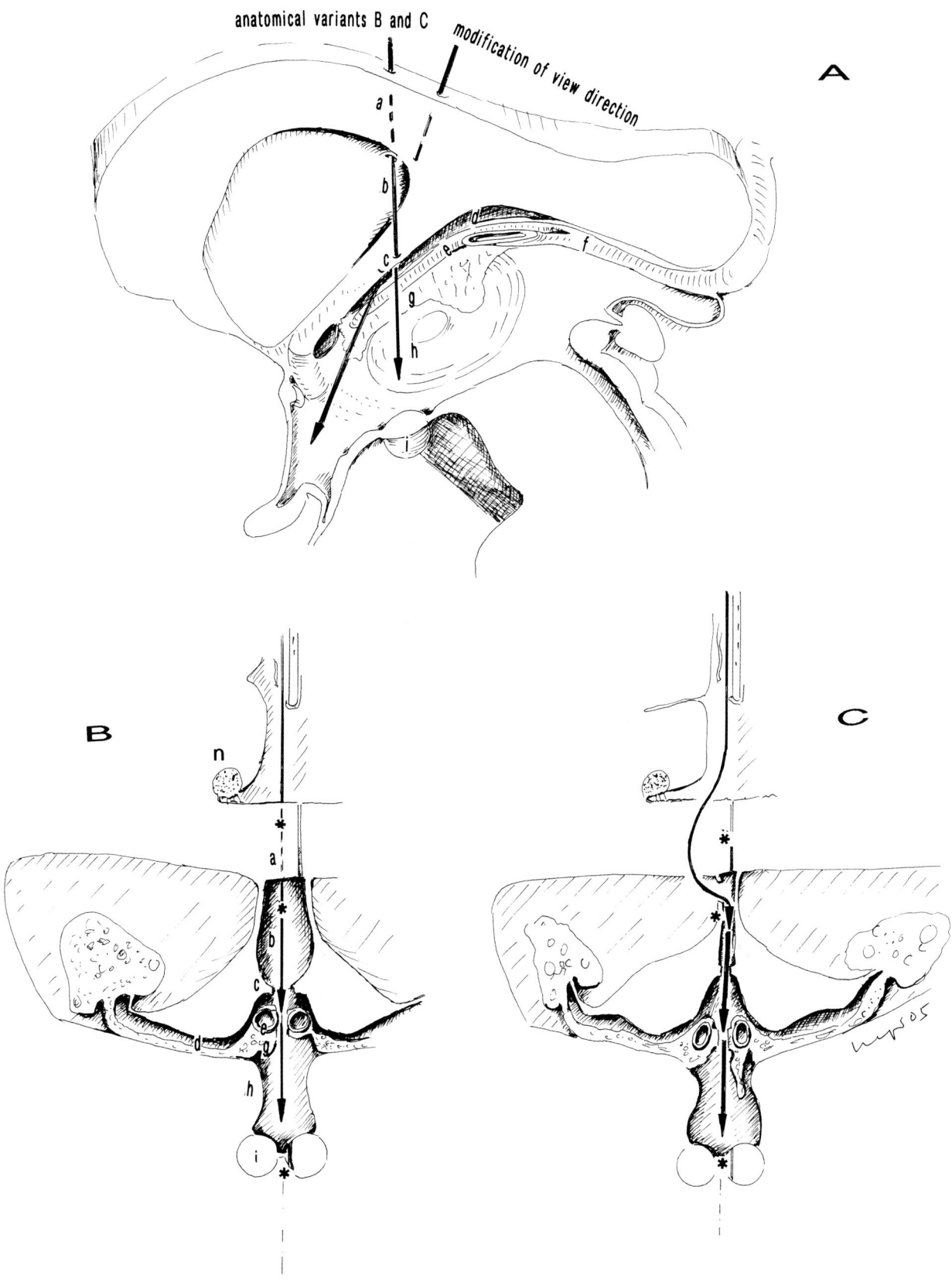

anatomical variants B and C

modification of view direction

* neuronavigatory landmarks

Fig. 34

Addendum for Fig. 33

D   Routes to the anterior and posterior target areas of the 3rd ventricle by incision of Commissura fornicis. Midline not defined by Cavum septi pellucidi

E   In prefixed Fornices, Commissura fornicis is wide, and Crura fornicis are far distant from each other. Incision of Commissura fornicis would less endanger Crura fornicis than at a normal (= narrow) commissure

F   Long variant of V. magna (Galeni). An approach crossing Fissura transversa between Vv. cerebri intt. Is not possible. V. magna (Galeni) defines the midline. It must be moved to the side for opening the roof (= Velum interpositum) of the 3rd ventricle

Abbreviations

a	Corpus callosum
b	Septum pellucidum
c'	Commissura fornicis
d	Fissura transversa cerebri
e	V. cerebri int.
f	V. magna (Galeni) (enclosed by Velum interpositum)
f'	choroid branches (enclosed by Velum interpositum)
g	Velum interpositum, enclosing the galenic vein
h	Thalamus, medial surface
i	Corp. mamillare
j	Lamina terminalis (close to Recessus opt.)
k	Columna fornicis, Pars tecta
l	Crus fornicis
m	Splenium corporis callosi
n	Area dentata, begin of striae
n'	Area dentata

FIG. 34

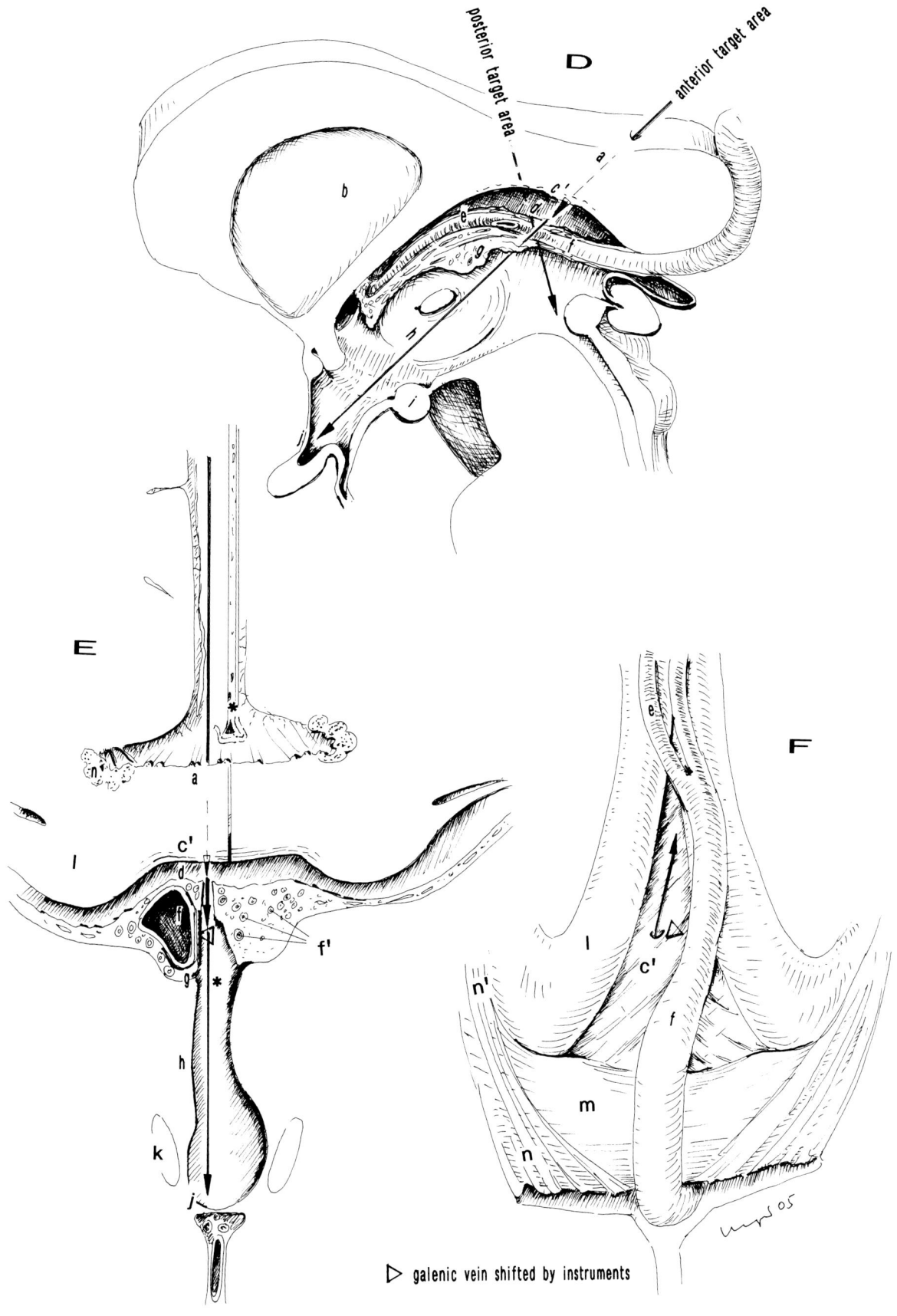

▷ galenic vein shifted by instruments

Fig. 35

Cavum Vergae is a dilatation of Cavum septi pellucidi or its posterior segment

A   At Cavum Vergae, all areas of the 3rd ventricle can be reached
B   Surgical approach for the posterior area of the 3rd ventricle
C   Surgical approach for the anterior area of the 3rd ventricle

For different length of the galenic vein see Fig. 34

Light arrows: Further modifications of surgical approaches

FIG. 35

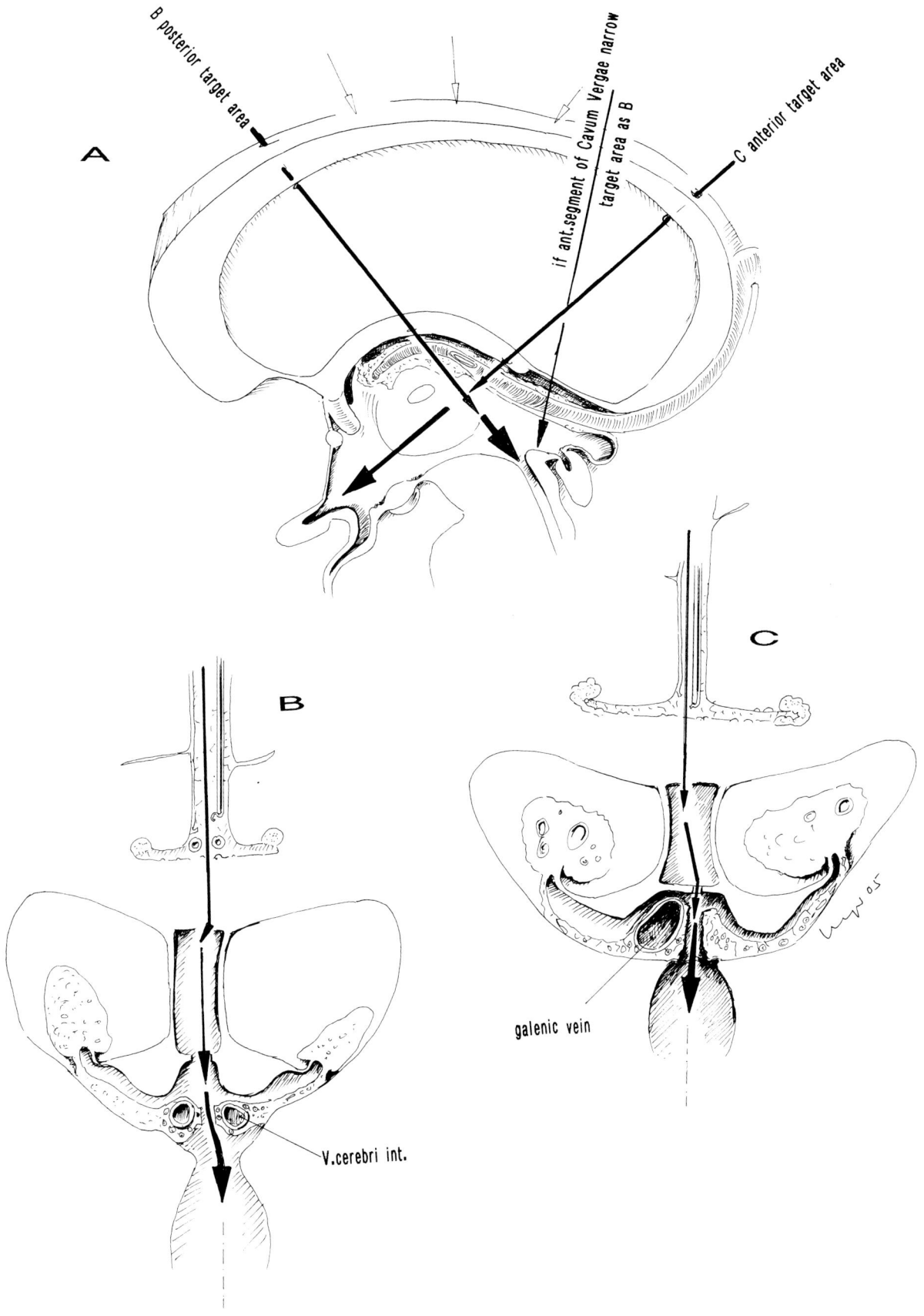

B posterior target area

if ant.segment of Cavum Vergae narrow target area as B

C anterior target area

A

C

B

V.cerebri int.

galenic vein

Fig. 36

Common variants of Vv. cerebri intt., V. magna (Galeni) and V. septi pellucidi

A   V. ventriculi lat. directa, combined with a shortening of V. magna (Galeni), and a widening of the distance between (light arrows) Vv. cerebri intt.

A'   Addendum for A

C   V. ventriculi lateralis directa. Oblique presentation of an fMRT. Normal individual

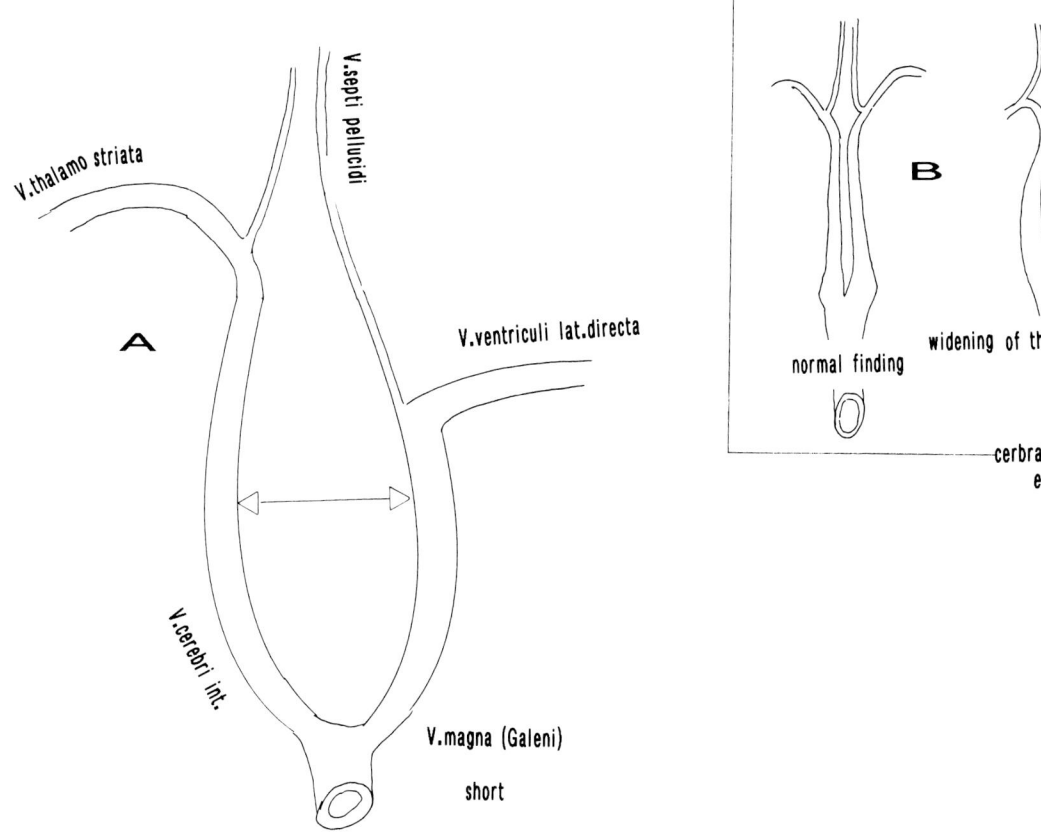

V.thalamo striata

V.septi pellucidi

A

V.ventriculi lat.directa

V.cerebri int.

V.magna (Galeni)

short

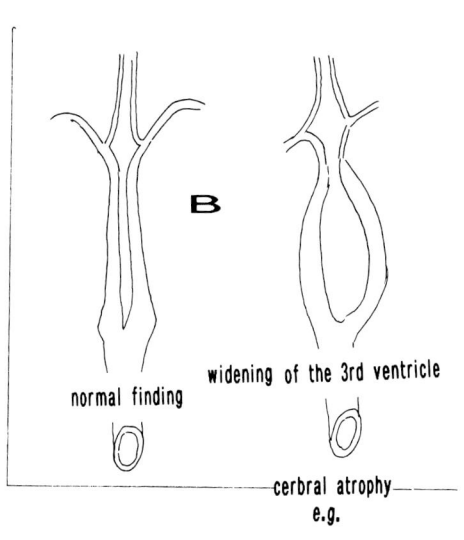

B

normal finding

widening of the 3rd ventricle

cerbral atrophy
e.g.

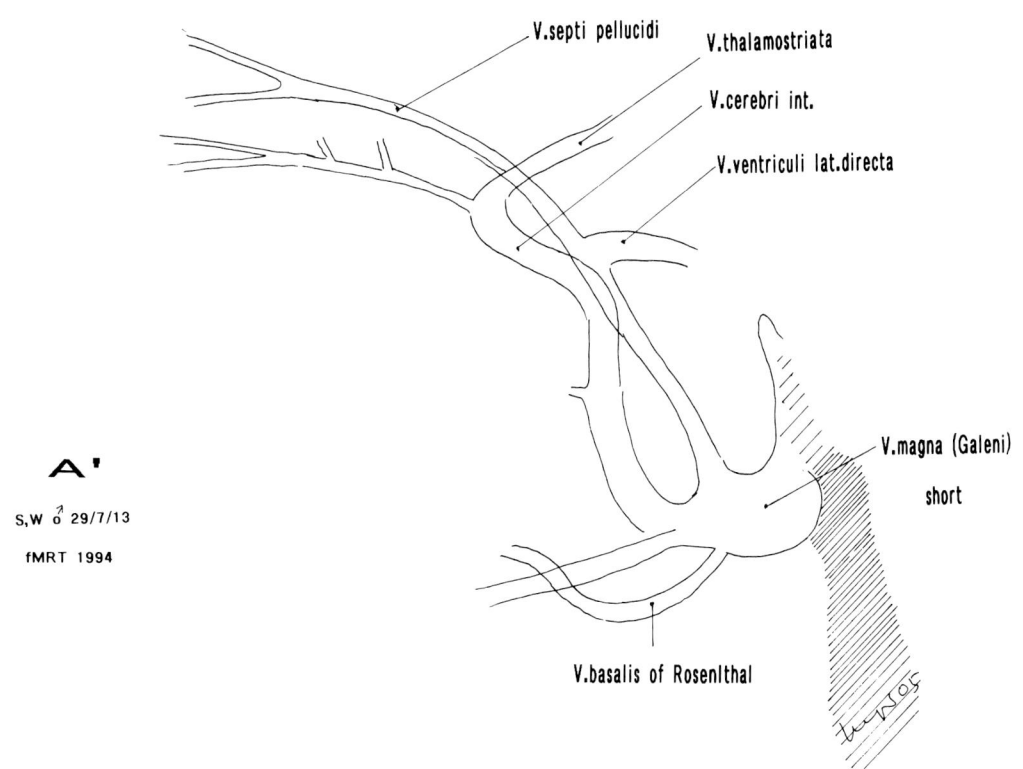

V.septi pellucidi

V.thalamostriata

V.cerebri int.

V.ventriculi lat.directa

V.magna (Galeni)

short

A'

S,W ♂ 29/7/13

fMRT 1994

V.basalis of Rosenlthal

Supracerebellar approaches to the 3rd ventricle and surrounding cisterns
(Krause-Yasargil) (Figs. 37 to 47)

Fig. 37

Principles of surgical approaches

A Overview
– Cerebellodorsal subdural approach, until the anterior medial margin of the arachnoid fold of the tentorial edge is reached (1st step)
– Transversal incision of the outer arachnoid layer between Culmen cerebelli and the tentorial edge. Loosening of cisternal adhesions and vessels, until Recessus suprapinealis is reached (2nd step)
– Incision and widening of the incised Recessus suprapinealis, introduction of the endoscope into the 3rd ventricle (3rd step)

B Problematic areas of this surgical approach
V. magna (Galeni)
Pinealis-Habenula-complex and adjacent structures

FIG. 37

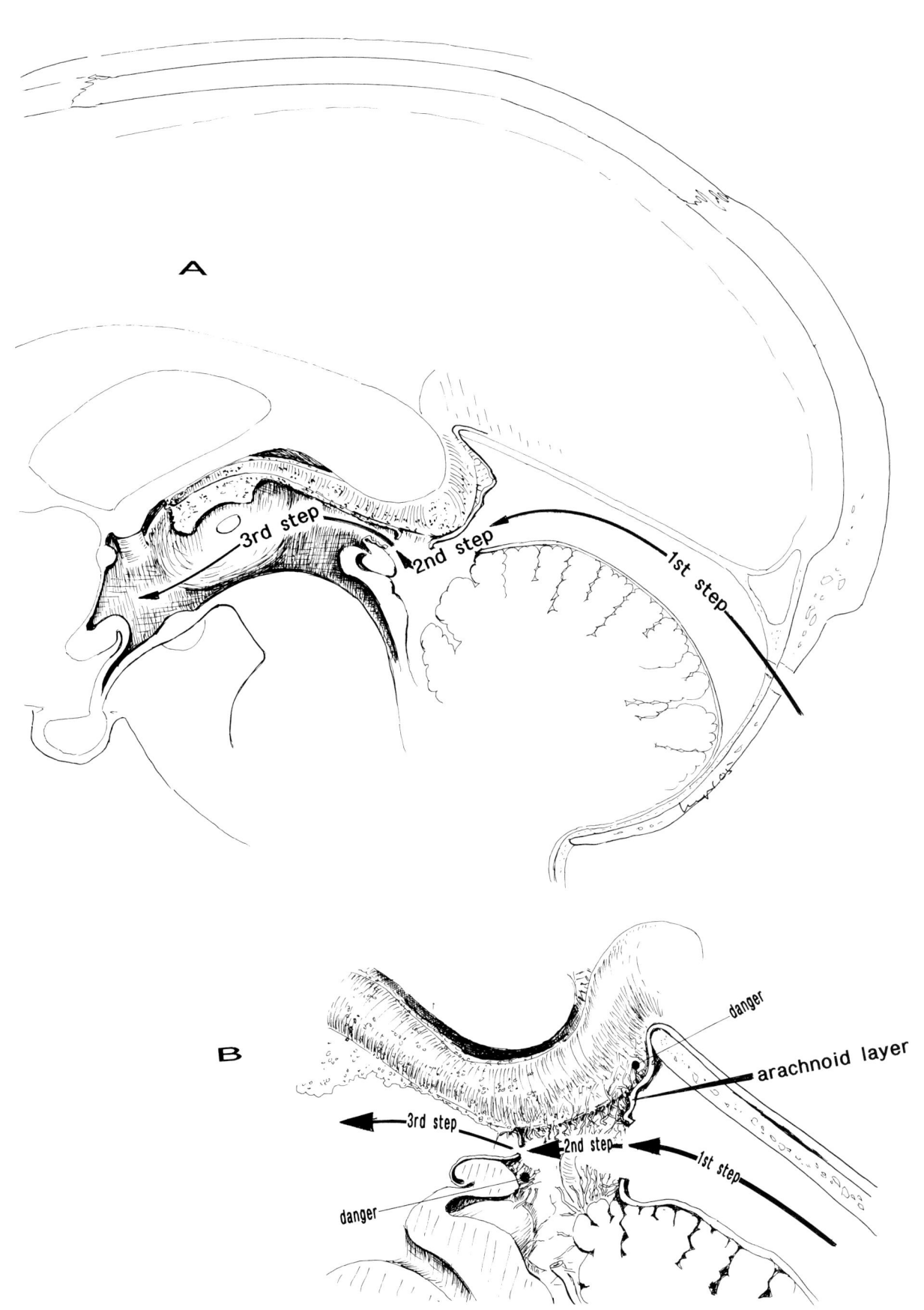

Details (Figs. 38 to 42)

Fig. 38

Positioning on the operation table

A   Anatomical sketch for planning strategies, if a horizontal approach is desired

B   Surgical routes, schematical drawing
Dotted line: orbito-meatal level

FIG. 38

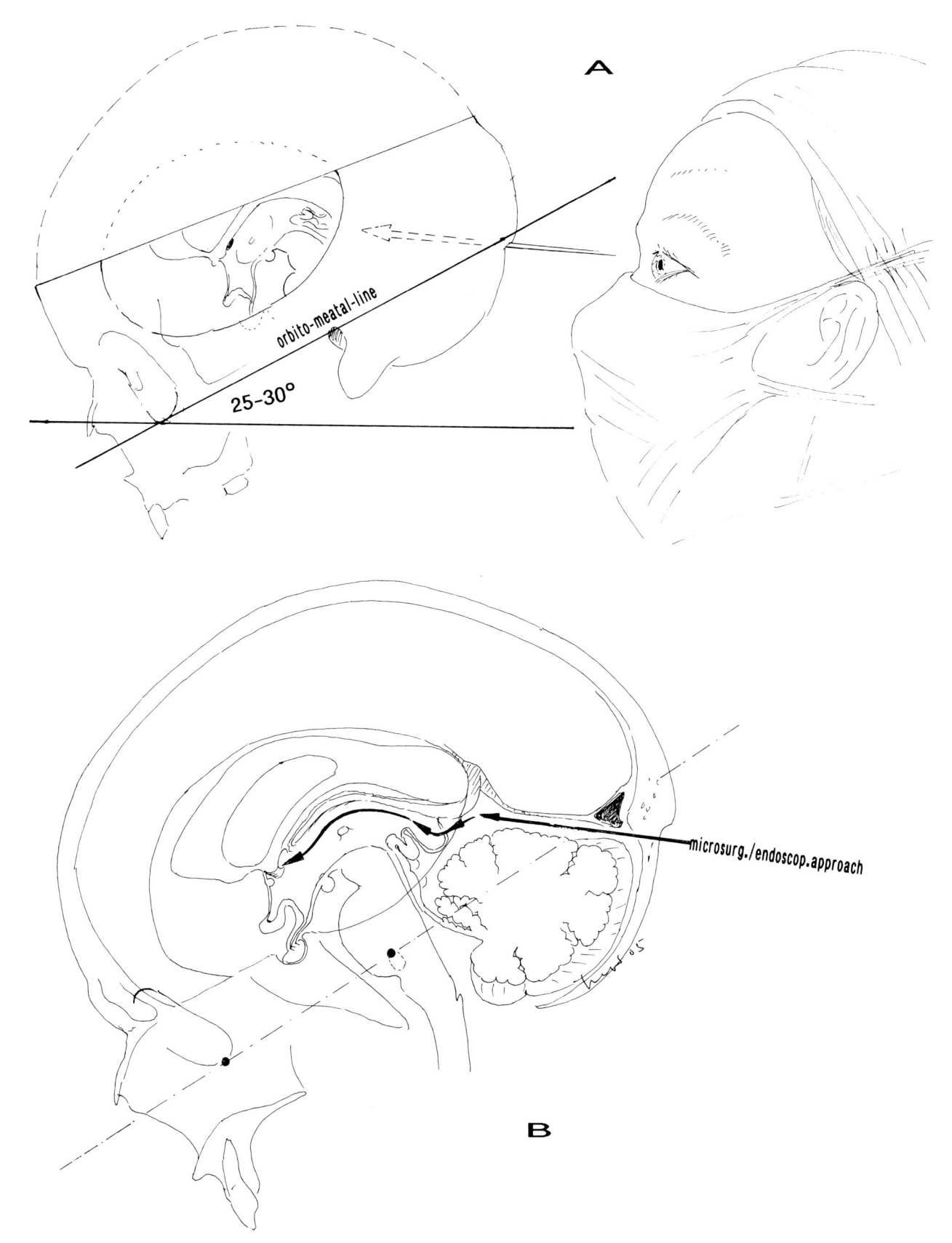

A

orbito-meatal-line

25-30°

microsurg./endoscop.approach

B

Fig. 39

Avoiding bridging veins

Surgical approaches may depend on variants of bridging veins

A   medial location of bridging veins (common type). Here the approach may begin dorsolaterally (lateral arrows). A midline approach, combined with craniotomy across the midline, can be carried out, if there are no hindering bridging veins

B   Bridging veins far laterally (less than 40%). Medial approaches necessary (arrows)

C and D According to A and B. Fine midline veins must be interrupted in the depth. In both approaches, the medial and the lateral approach, Culmen can be softly pushed down. The shifting of Culmen should be minimal, because there is danger for compression of the brainstem. Surgery should be continued by endoscope and not by microsurgery

E and F Before and after shifting of Culmen. Note extension of the arachnoid layer between the edge of Tentorium and Culmen (Transition of supratentorial and infratentorial Arachnoidea)

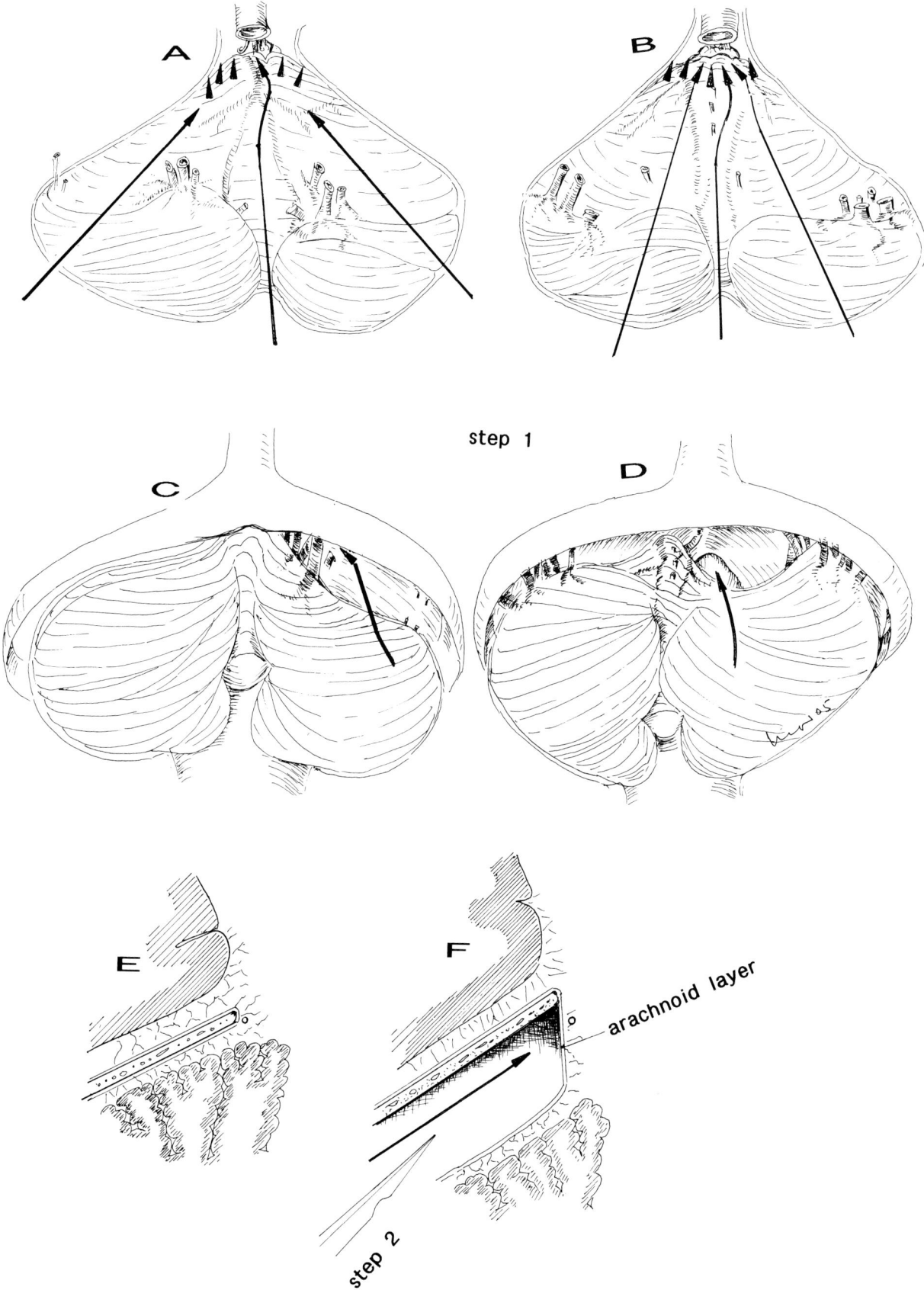

step 1

step 2

arachnoid layer

Avoiding V. magna (Galeni), Corpus pineale, area of Aquaeductus and surrounding structures (Figs. 40 to 42)

Fig. 40

– Opening of the outer arachnoid layer, loosening of trabeculae and vessels of Cisterna tecti (and Cisternae ambientes, if necessary), presentation of V. magna (Galeni), Tectum and Corpus pineale, until Recessus suprapinealis is reached (step 2)
– Presentation, opening and widening of the opening of Recessus suprapinealis (step 3)
– Inspection of the 3rd ventricle (step 4)

G   For understanding H
H   Surgical topography, overview (anatomical model)

Abbreviations
a   Tentorium (transection)
a'   edge of Tentorium (covered by the outer Arachnoidea)
b   Culmen
c   V. (Vv.) supraculminalis(es), V. (Vv.) cerebellaris(es) praecentralis(es) – singular, double or multiple veins –
d   Colliculus sup.
e   Commissura post.
f   Corpus pineale
g   Recessus suprapinealis
h   adhesions of the galenic vein and the outer arachnoid layer
i   N. trochlearis
j   V. magna (Galeni)
k   Vv. tecti
l   choroid arteries
m   as k, Baumgartner's loop close to V. basalis Rosenthal and Pulvinar thalami

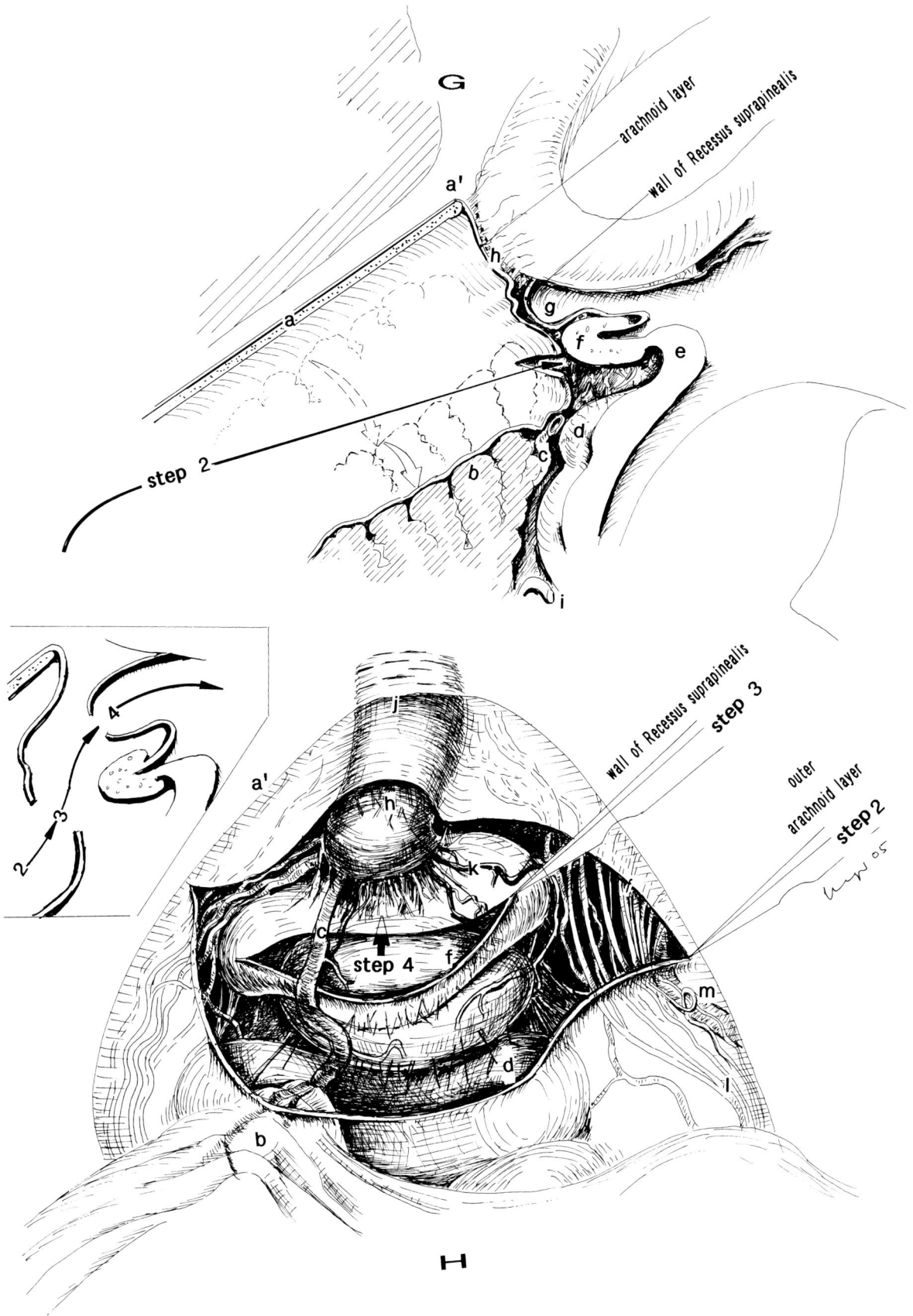

G

arachnoid layer

wall of Recessus suprapinealis

a'

h

g

f

e

a

d

c

b

i

step 2

step 2

step 3

wall of Recessus suprapinealis

outer arachnoid layer

a'

j

h

k

c

step 4

f

m

d

l

b

H

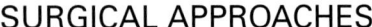

Fig. 41

Intraoperative injury to V. magna (Galeni) at incision of the outer arachnoid layer

Incision of the outer arachnoid layer too far dorsal and in the midline. Often the outer arachnoid layer is not transparent, and the vein is not to be identified before the arachnoid layer is incised
The horizontal incision of the outer arachnoid layer may begin close to Culmen and besides the midline (step 2, see Fig. 40)

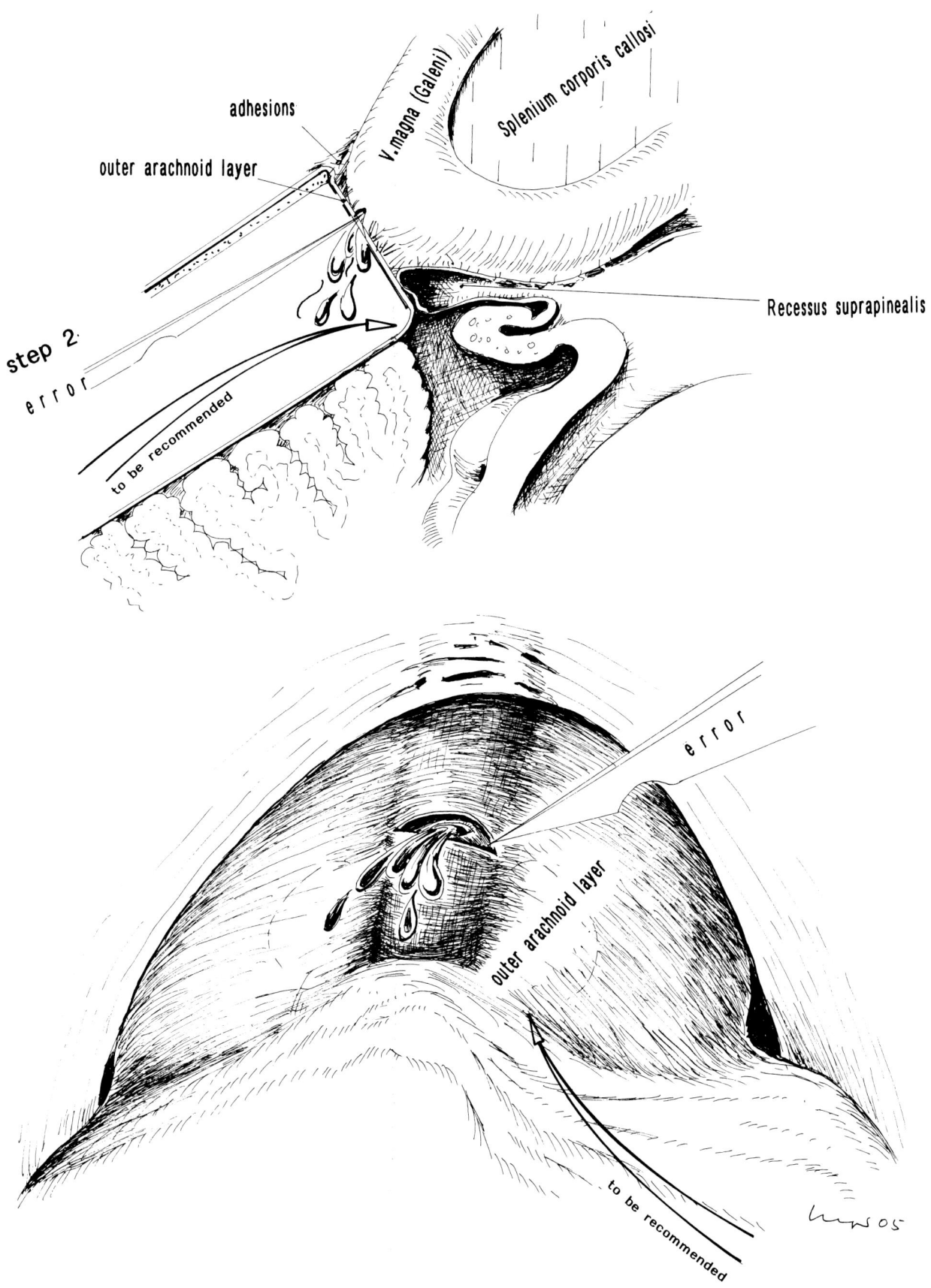

adhesions

outer arachnoid layer

V. magna (Galeni)

Splenium corporis callosi

Recessus suprapinealis

step 2

error

to be recommended

error

outer arachnoid layer

to be recommended

Fig. 42

Danger for damage of Corpus pineale and its adjacent structures

A   Surgical approach (arrow) correct, crossing the opened Recessus suprapinealis
A' Surgical topography according to A

B   Surgical approach (arrow) via falsa. The approach crosses an artificial gap between Corpus pineale and Commissura post.
        Corpus pineale is adherent with the galenic-vein-Recessus-suprapinealis-complex, because the loosening of Corpus pineale from dorsal adhesions was not sufficient.
B' Surgical topography according to B

Abbreviations
a   Corpus pineale
b   Recessus pinealis
c   Commissura habenularum
d   Commissura post.
e   Aquaeductus
f   Habenula
g   Colliculus sup.
h   Lobulus centralis cerebelli

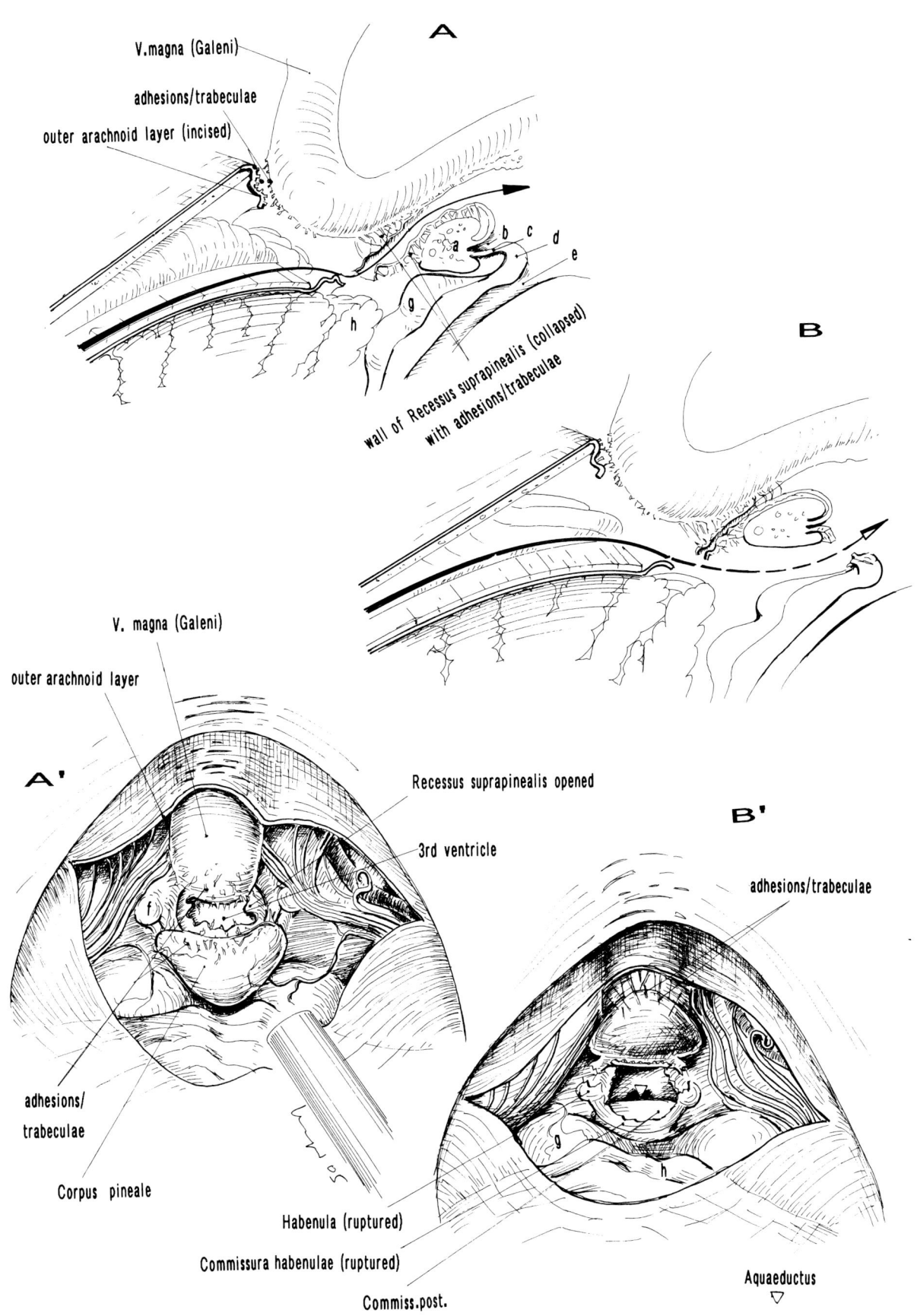

A

V.magna (Galeni)

adhesions/trabeculae

outer arachnoid layer (incised)

a b c d e

g

h

wall of Recessus suprapinealis (collapsed)
with adhesions/trabeculae

B

V. magna (Galeni)

outer arachnoid layer

A'

Recessus suprapinealis opened

3rd ventricle

B'

adhesions/trabeculae

f

g

h

adhesions/
trabeculae

Corpus pineale

Habenula (ruptured)

Commissura habenulae (ruptured)

Commiss.post.

Aquaeductus
▽

Figs. 43 to 47

Target areas of the 3rd ventricle and of Fissura transversa, special anatomical and surgical aspects

Fig. 43

Overview

A   Target area 3rd ventricle
B   Target area Fissura transversa

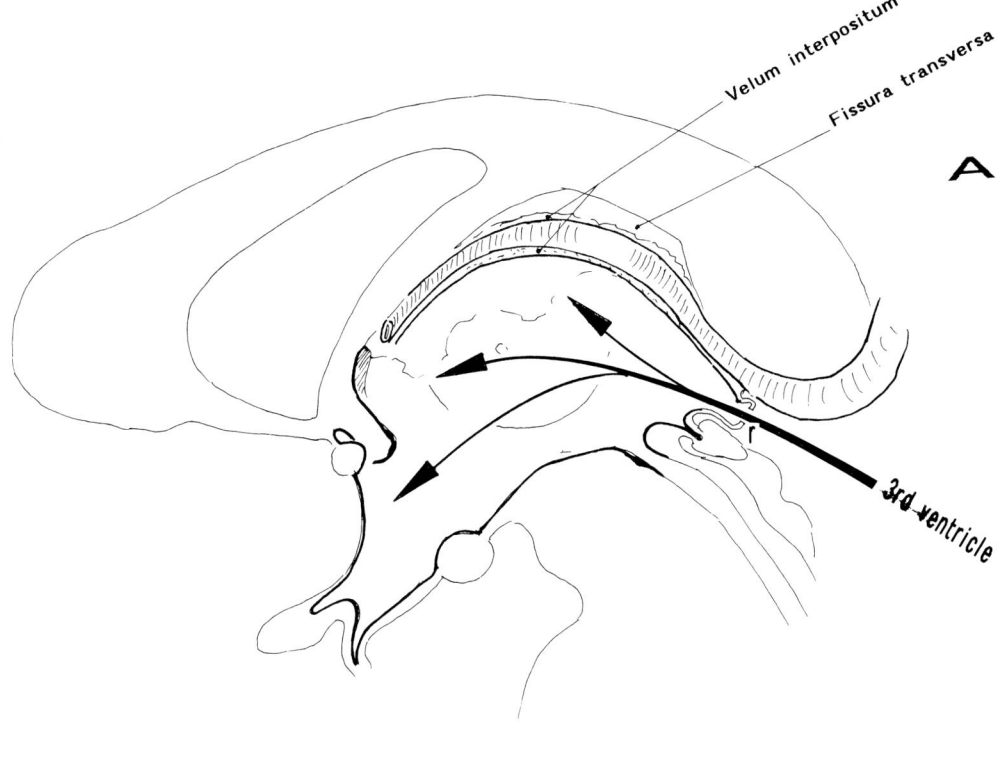

Velum interpositum

Fissura transversa

A

r

3rd ventricle

r

Recessus suprapinealis, opened

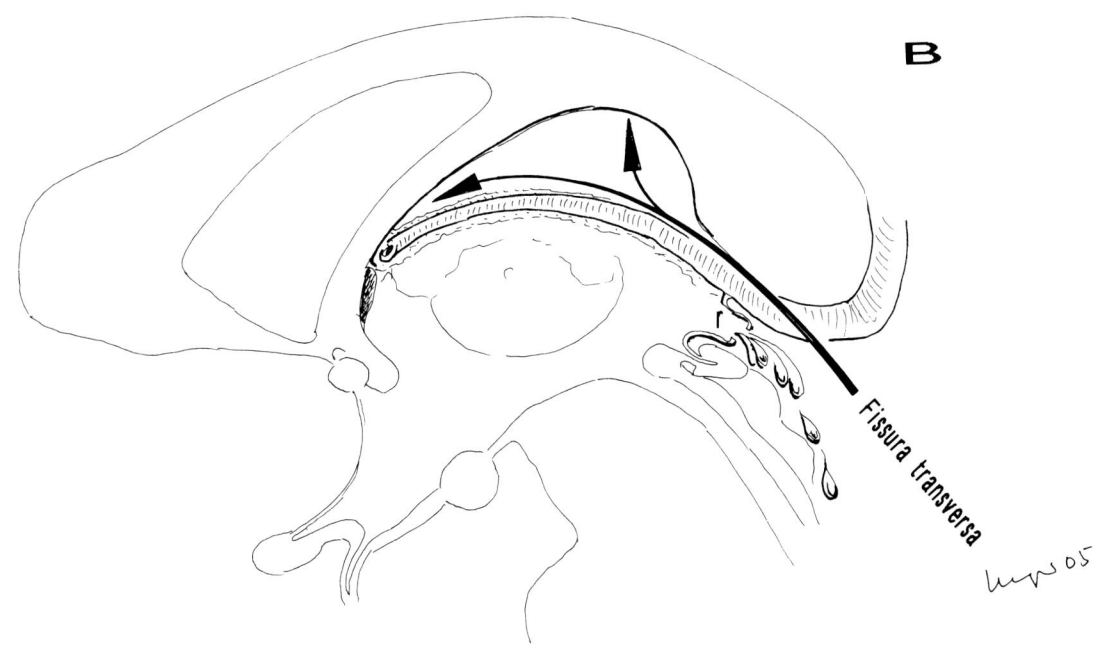

B

r

Fissura transversa

Fig. 44

Both spaces – Fissura transversa and 3rd ventricle, coronal presentation

A   Topogram for B
B   Coronal presentation of both spaces

FIG. 44

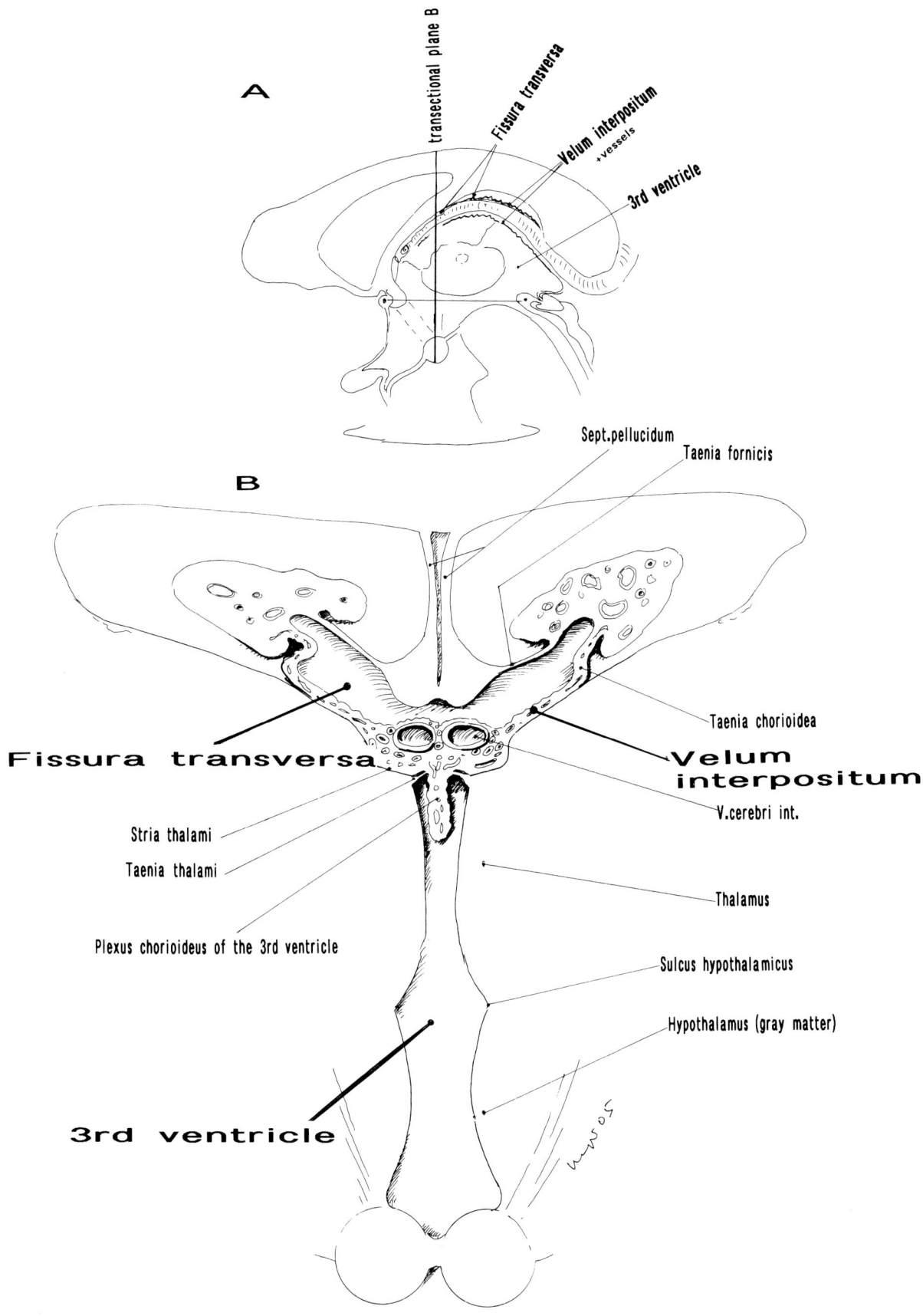

A

transectional plane B

Fissura transversa

Velum interpositum
+ vessels

3rd ventricle

B

Sept.pellucidum

Taenia fornicis

Fissura transversa

Taenia chorioidea

Velum interpositum

Stria thalami

V.cerebri int.

Taenia thalami

Thalamus

Plexus chorioideus of the 3rd ventricle

Sulcus hypothalamicus

Hypothalamus (gray matter)

3rd ventricle

Fig. 45

Surgical approach to the 3rd ventricle, anatomical presentations

A   Surgical routes using endoscopy

B   Anatomical approach after cutting of Recessus suprapinealis and loosening of Velum interpositum from its Taeniae. Fornices dissected. The 3rd ventricle is opened (light arrows)

B' Anatomical panoramic view. For view directions see B
Velum interpositum loosened and elevated in a dorsal direction, as it is presented in Fig. 46 B

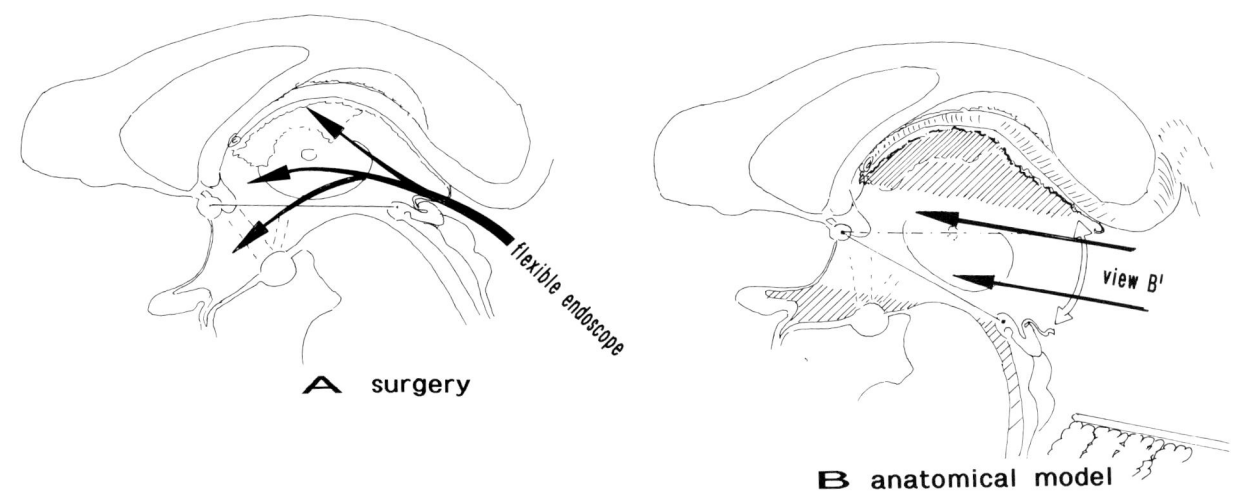

flexible endoscope

A surgery

view B'

B anatomical model

a
b
c
d
e
f
g
h
i
j
k
l
Columnae fornicis
For.interventriculare (Monroi)
insertions of Velum interpositum
Taenia chorioidea
Taenia thalami
Stria terminalis
Lamina affixa
Stria thalami
Habenula
Commiss.habenularum
wall of Recess.suprapin.,residual

B'
anatomical model

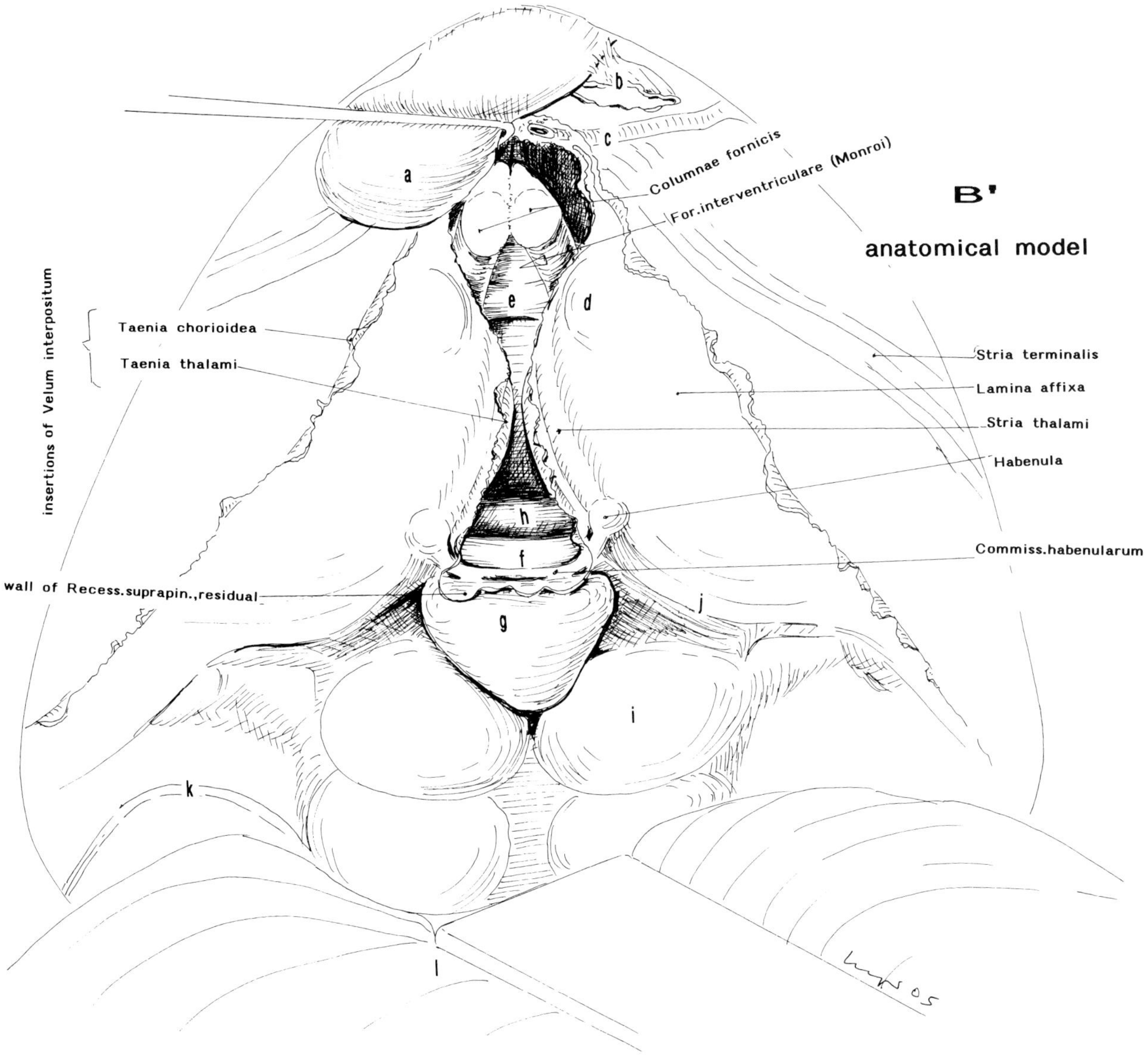

Fig. 46

Surgical approach to Fissura transversa, anatomical presentations

A   Velum interpositum is interposed
      – between 3rd ventricle/both thalami and Fissura transversa

      Anatomical shifting in a dorsal direction may be done after cutting of its basal
      connections:
      – Recessus suprapinealis (a)
      – Taeniae thalami, see B (h)
      – Taeniae chorioideae, see B (i)
        Light arrows: Wide opening of the anatomical approach for Fissura transversa

B   Velum interpositum, view from a basal direction, for presentation of its basal
      connections after dissection. Its small medial segment builts the roof of the 3rd
      ventricle, its wide lateral areas cover the dorsal medial segments of Thalami, as
      presented in C

C   Fissura tranversa wide opened. Its roof is formed by both Fornices and Commis-
      sura fornicis (o)
      Its bottom consists of Velum interpositum, which encloses chorioid vessels, inner
      cerebral veins and V. basalis (Rosenthal)
      The anterior point of its trigonal shape is the posterior wall of the foramen of
      Monro. The wall is connected with the anterior medial segment of both Thalami
      and with Columnae fornicis.
C'   Addendum for C

Abbreviations
a   Recessus suprapinealis
b   Columnae fornicis
c   Vv. cerebri intt.
d   V. basalis (Rosenthal
e   Aa. chorioideae postt.
f   For. interventriculare (Monroi)
g   Lamina affixa thalami
h   Taeniae thalami
i   Taeniae chorioideae
j   Stria terminalis
k   V. thalamostriata
l   Corpus pineale
m   Colliculus sup.
n   N. trochlearis
o   Commissura fornicis

FIG. 46

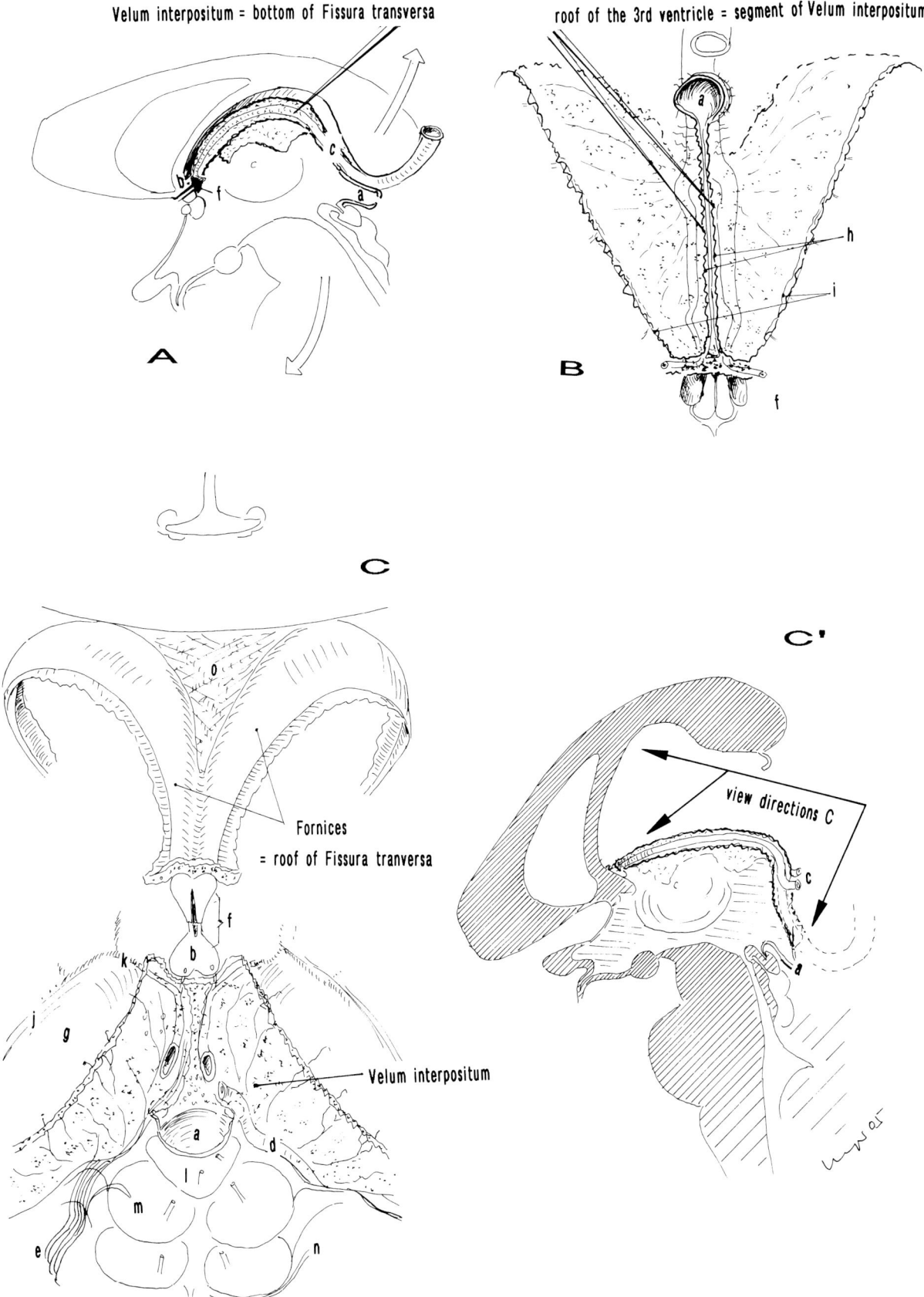

Velum interpositum = bottom of Fissura transversa

A

roof of the 3rd ventricle = segment of Velum interpositum

B

C

Fornices
= roof of Fissura tranversa

Velum interpositum

C'

view directions C

Fig. 47

Surgical approaches to the 3rd ventricle and to Fissura transversa

A   Fissura transversa, panoramic view. Combination of different surgical presentations
B   3rd ventricle, panoramic view. Combination of different surgical presentations
C   Addendum for A and B

Abbreviations
a   Crus fornicis
b   Commissura fornicis
c   Taenia fornicis
d   Corpus fornicis
d'   Columna fornicis
e   Fissura chorioidea
f   Velum interpositum
g   V. cerebri int., enclosd by f
h   post. chor. arteries, medial group
i   V. basalis (Rosenthal
j   V. magna (Galeni)
k   Habenula
(k) as k, projection
l   Commissura anterior
m   Commissura posterior
n   Thalamus
o   Foramen interventriculare (Monroi)
p   Lamina terminalis
q   Colliculus sup.
r   medial and lateral group of choroid arteries
s   Corpus pineale

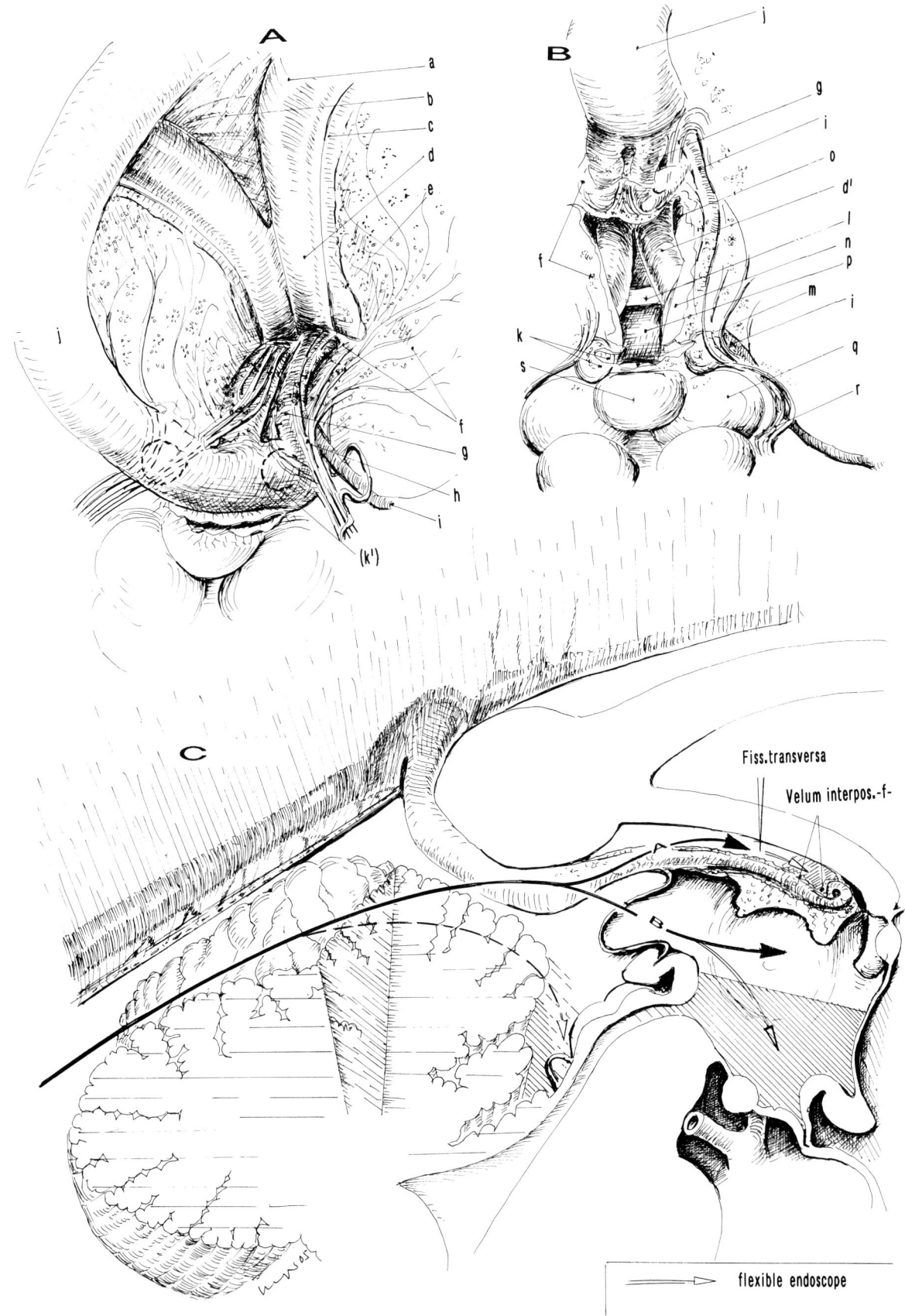

A

a
b
c
d
e
j
f
g
h
i
(k')

B

j
g
i
o
d'
l
n
p
m
i
q
r
f
k
s

C

Fiss.transversa
Velum interpos.-f-

flexible endoscope

References

Overview

Anatomical Basis

Browder J, Kaplan HA (1975) Cerebral dural sinuses and their tributaries, Thomas, Springfield I11

Browder J, Kaplan HA (1976) Cerebral dural sinuses and their tributaries. Ch C Thomas, Springfield I11

Corrales M, Torrealba G (1976) The third ventricle. Normal anatomy and changes in some pathological conditions. Neuroradiology 11: 271–277

Dimond SJ, Scammell RE, Brouwers EYM et al (1977) Functions of the centre section (trunk) of the corpus callosum in man. Brain 100: 543–562

Duvernoy HM (1978) Human Breinstem vessels. Springer, Berlin Heidelberg New York Tokyo

Gazzaniga MS, Freedman H (1973) Observations on visual processes after posterior callosal section. Neurology (Minneap) 23: 1126–1130

Gordon HW, Bogen JE, Speery RW (1971) Absence of deconnexion syndrome in two patients with partial section of the neocommissures. Brain 94: 327–336

Heilman KM, Sypert GW (1977) Korsakoff's syndrome resulting from bilateral fornix lesions. Neurology (NY) 27: 490–493

Huang YP, Wolf BS (1966) Precentral cerebellar vein in angiography. Acta Radiol (Stockh) 5: 250–262

Jeeves MA, Simpson DA, Geffen G (1979) Functional consequences of the transcallosal removal of intraventricular tumours. J Neurol Neurosurg Psychiatry 42: 134–142

Kaplan see Browder and Kaplan

Krause F (1938) Die spezielle Chirurgie der Gehirnerkrankungen in 3 Bänden, I Band, S 16–18

Lang J (1981) Klinische Anatomie des Kopfes. Springer, Berlin Heidelberg New York Tokyo

Marino R (1976) The anterior cerebral artery: I. Anatomoradiological study of its cortical territories. Surg Neurol 5: 81–87

McRae DL, Castorina G (1963) Variations in corpus callosum, septum pellucidum and fornix, and their effect on the encephalogram and cerebral angiography. Acta Radiol 1: 872–880

Milhorat TH, Baldwin M (1966) A technique for surgical exposure of the cerebral midline. Experimental transcallosal microdissection. J Neurosurg 24: 687–691

Plets C (1969) The arterial blood supply and architecture of the posterior wall of the third ventricle. Acta Neurochir (Wien) 21

Retzius G (1900) Biologische Untersuchungen, neue Folge 9, Tafel XII. Gustav Fischer (see Corrales and Torrealba), Jena

Salamon G (1971) Atlas de la vascularisation artérielle du cerveau chez l'homme. Atlas of the arteries of the human brain. Sandoz, Paris

Salamon G, Huang YP (1976) Radiologic anatomy of the brain. Springer, Berlin Heidelberg New York Tokyo

Seeger W (1978) Atlas of topographical anatomy of the brain and surrounding structures. Springer, Wien New York

Seeger W (2003) Standard variants of the skull and brain, pp 242ff, 254ff, 260, 266ff, 276ff, 288, 290. Springer, Wien New York

Spalteholz W (1906/7) Handatlas der Anatomie des Menschen, 3. Bd. Hirzel, Leipzig, p 636

Sperry RW, Gazzaniga MS, Bogen JE (1969) Interhemispheric relationships. The neocortical commissures; syndromes of hemisphere disconnection. In: Vinken PJ, Bruyn GW (eds) Disorders of speech, perception, and symbolic behaviour. Handbook of clinical neurology, vol. 4. North-Holland, Amsterdam, pp 273–290

Sweet WH, Talland GA, Ervin FR (1959) Loss of recent memory following section of the fornix. Trans Am Neurol Assoc 84: 76–82

Stephan H (1975) Allocortex. In: Bargmann W (ed) Handbuch der mikroskopischen Anatomie des Menschen, IV, Nervensystem. Springer, Berlin Heidelberg New York Tokyo

Stephens RB, Stilwell DL (1969) Arteries and veins of the human brain. Ch C Thomas, Springfield I11

Winston KR, Cavazzuti V, Arkins T (1979) Absence of neurological and behavioral abnormalities after anterior transcallosal operation for third ventricular lesions. Neurosurgery 4: 386–393

Woolsey RM, Nelson JS (1975) Asymptomatic destruction of the fornix in man. Arch Neurol 32: 566–568

Zaidel D, Sperry KW (1974) Memory impairment after commissurotomy in man. Brain 97: 263–272

Zuleger S, Staubesand J (1977) Atlas of the central nervous system in sectional planes. Urban & Schwarzenberg, Baltimore-Munich

Surgical Approaches

Abbot R (2004) History of neuroendoscopy. Neurosurg Clin N Am 15: 1–7

Antunes JL, Muraszko K, Quest DO, Carmel PW (1982) Surgical strategies in the management of tumours of the anterior third ventricle. In: Brock M (ed) Modern neurosurgery. Springer, Berlin Heidelberg New York Tokyo

Apuzzo MLJ (1982) Transcallosal interfornical exposure of lesions of the third ventricle. In: Schmidek HH, Sweet WH (eds) Operative neurosurgical techniques. Grune and Stratton, New York, pp 585–594

Apuzzo MLJ (1987) Surgery of the third ventricle. Williams & Wilkins, Baltimore London Los Angeles Sydney

Apuzzo MLJ, Chikovani OK, Gott PS, Teng EL, Zee CS, Giannotta SL, Weiss MH (1982) Transcallosal, interfornical approaches for lesions affecting the third ventricle: surgical considerations and consequences. Neurosurgery 10: 547–554

Bengochea FG, De La Torre O, Esquivel O et al (1959) The section of the fornix in the surgical treatment of certain epilepsies. Trans Am Neurol Assoc 79: 176–178

Browder J, Kaplan HA (1975) Cerebral dural sinuses and their tributaries, Thomas, Springfield I11

Dandy WE (1922) Diagnosis, localization and removal of tumours of the third ventricle. Bull Johns Hopkins Hosp 33: 188–189

Dandy WE (1933) Benign tumours in the third ventricle of the brain; Diagnosis and treatment. Thomas Ch C, Springfield I11

Foerster O (1932) Über das operative Vorgehen bei Operationen der Vierhügelgegend. Zbl ges Neurol Psychiat 61: 457–459

Geffen G, Walsh A, Simpson D, Jeeves M (1980) Comparison of the effects of transcortical and transcallosal removal of intraventricular tumours. Brain 103: 773–788

Gerzeni M, Cohen AR (1998) Advances in endoscopic neurosurgery. AORN J 67: 957

Grant JA, McLone DG (1997) Third ventriculostomy: a review. Surg Neurol 47: 210–212

Harris LW (1994) Endoscopic techniques in neurosurgery. Microsurgery 15: 541–546

Harris AE, Hadjipanayis CG, Lunsford LD, Lunsford AK, Kassam AB (2005) Microsurgical removal of intraventricular lesions using endoscopic visualization and stereotactic guidance. Neurosurgery 56: 125–132

Hellwig D, Bauer BL (1992) Minimally invasive neurosurgery by means of ultrathin endoscopes. Acta Neurochir [Suppl] 54: 63–68

Hellwig D, Grotenhuis JA, Tiracotai W, Riegel T, Schulte DM, Bauer BL, Bertalanffy H (2005) Endoscopic third ventriculostomy for obstructive hydrocephalus. Neurosurg Rev 28: 1–34

Hirsch JF, Zouaoui A, Renier D, Pierre-Kahn A (1979) A new surgical approach to the third ventricle with interruption of the striothalamic vein. Acta Neurochir (Wien) 47: 135–147

Hirschowitz BJ (1988) The development and application of fiberoptic endoscopy. Cancer 61 (10): 1935–1941

Hirschowitz BJ, Peters CW, Curtiss LE, Pollard HM (1958) Demonstration of a new gastroscope, the "Fiberscope" Gastroenterology 35: 50–53

Huewel NM, Perneczky A, Urban V (1993) Neuroendoscopic techniques in operativ treatment of syringomyelia Acta Neurochir (Wien) 123: 216

Jho HD, Carrau RL, McLaughlin MR, Somaza SC (1997) Endoscopic transshenoidal resection of a large chordoma in the posterior fossa. Acta Neurochir (Wien) 139: 343–347

Jaikumar S, Kim DH, Kam AC (2002) History of minimally invasive spine surgery. Neurosurgery 51: 1–14

Kaplan see Browder and Kaplan

Kassam A, Horowitz M, Welch W, Sclabassi R, Carrau R, Snyderman C, Hirsch B (2005) The role of endoscolpic assisted microneurosurgery (image fusion technology) in the performance of neurosurgical procedures. Minim Invasive Neurosurg 48: 191–196

King TT (1979) Removal of intraventricular craniopharyngiomas through the lamina terminalis. Acta Neurochir (Wien) 45: 277–286

Krause F (1926) Operative Freilegung der Vierhügel nebst Beobachtungen über Hirndruck und Dekompression. Zbl Chir 53: 2812–2819

Landolt AM (2001) History of pituitary surgery from the technical aspect. Neurosurg Clin N Am 12: 37–viii

Lang J (1981) Klinische Anatomie des Kopfes. Springer, Berlin Heidelberg New York Tokyo

Le Gars D, Lejeune JP (2000) Introduction and history of surgery of the third ventricle. Neurochirurgie 46: 137–140

Long DM, Chou SN (1973) Transcallosal removal of craniopharyngiomas within the third ventricle. J Neurosurg 39: 563–567

Long DM, Leibrock L (1980) The transcallosal approach to the anterior ventricular system and its application in the therapy of craniopharyngioma. Clin Neurosurg C N S 27: 160–168

Marino R (1976) The anterior cerebral artery: I. Anatomico-radiological study of its cortical territories. Surg Neurol 5: 81–87

Mixter WJ (1923) Ventriculoscopy and puncture of the floor of the third ventricle. Boston Med Surg J 188: 277–278

Olinger CP, Ohlhaber RL (1974) Eighteen – gauge microscopic – telescopic needle endoscope and electrode channel: potential clinical and research application. Surg Neurol 2: 151–160

Perneczky G, Loyoddin M, Markowitsch MM (2000) Intrakranielle Neuroendoskopie, J Neurolog, Neurochir Psychiatrie 1: 22–26

Poppen JL (1960) An atlas of neurosurgical techniques. WB Saunders Company, Philadelphia London

Retzius G (1900) Biologische Untersuchungen, neue Folge 9, Tafel XII. Gustav Fischer (see Corrales and Torrealba), Jena

Rhoton AL Jr, Yamamoto I, Peace DA (1981) Microsurgery of the third ventricle: part 2. Operative approaches. Neurosurgery 8: 357–373

Seeger W (1980) Microsurgery of the brain II. Springer, Wien New York, p 578ff

Seeger W (1984) Microsurgery of cerebral veins. Springer, Wien New York, pp 236, 302, 314ff

Seeger W (1985) Differential approaches in microsurgery of the brain. Springer, Wien New York, pp 6ff, 94, 98ff, 172, 248

Seeger W (1988) Anatomical dissections for use in neurosurgery, vol 2. Springer, Wien New York, pp 136ff, 246ff, 284ff

Seeger W (1990) Strategies of microsurgery in problematic brain areas – with special reference to NMR. pp 124ff, 172ff

Seeger W (1993) The microsurgical approaches to the target areas of the brain. Springer, Wien New York, pp 228ff, 234, 236ff, 270ff, 274ff

Seeger W (2000) Microanatomical aspects for neurosurgeons and neuroradiologists. Springer, Wien New York, pp 98, 134ff, 160, 164ff, 168

Seeger W, Zentner J (2002) Neuronavigation and neuroanatomy. Springer, Wien New York, pp 104ff, 174ff, 182fff, 206ff, 214ff, 256ff

Shucart WA, Stein BM (1978) Transcallosal approach to the anterior ventricular system. Neurosurgery 3: 339–343

Souweidane MM, Sandberg DI, Bilsky MH, Gutin PH (2000) Endoscopic biopsy for tumors of the third ventricle. Pediatr Neurosurg 33: 132–137

Suzuki J, Katakura R, Mori T (1984) Interhemispheric approach through the lamina terminalis to tumours of the anterior part of the third ventricle. Surg Neurol 22: 157–163

Schroeder HW, Niendorf WR, Gaab MR (2002) Complications of endoscopic third ventriculostomy. J Neurosurg 96: 1032–1040

Stefanov I, Stefanov A, Westman J (1996) A new method for transcutaneous coaxial neuroendoscopy. AnatEmbryol 194: 319–326

Stranjalis G, Sakas DE (2004) Letters to editor: minimal invasive neurosurgery 47: 258

Stein BM (1977) Transcallosal approach to third ventricular tumors. In: Schmidek HH, Sweet WH (eds) Current techniques in operative neurosurgery. Grune & Stratton, New York, pp 247–255

Uchiyama S, Hasegawa K, Homma T, Takahashi HE, Shimoji K (1998) Ultrafine flexible spinal endoscope (myeloscope) and discovery of an unreported subarachnoid lesion. Spine 23 (21): 2358–2362

Walker ML (2001) History of ventriculostomy. Neurosurg Clin N Am 12: 101–110, viii

Walker ML, MacDonald J, Wright LC (1992) The history of ventriculoscopy: where do we go from here? Pediatr Neurosurg 18: 218–223

Warnke JP, Koppert H, Bensch/Schreiter B, Dzelzitis J (2003) Thecaloscopy Part III. First clinical application. Minim Invas Neurosurg 46: 94–99

Warnke JP, Tschabitscher M, Nobels A (2001) Thecaloscopy. The Endoscopy of the lumbar subarachnoid. Space part I historical review and own cadaver studies. Minim Invas Neurosurg 2001 44: 61–64

Yamakawa K, Kondo T, Yoshioka M, Takakura as K (1992) Application of superfine fiberscope for endovasculoscopy, ventriculoscopy and myeloscopy. Acta Neurochir [Suppl] 54: 47–52

Yamamoto I, Rhoton AL JR, Peace DA (1981) Microsurgery of the third ventricle: part 1. Microsurgical anatomy. Neurosurgery 8: 334–356

Yaşargil MG et al (1976) Arteriovenous malformations of vein of Galen: microsurgical treatment. Surg Neurol 6: 195–200

Yaşargil MG, Jain KK, Antic J et al (1976) Arteriovenous malformations of the splenium of the corpus callosum: microsurgical treatment. Surg Neurol 5: 5–14

Subject Index

SpringerNeurosurgery

Wolfgang Seeger,
Josef Zentner

Neuronavigation
and Neuroanatomy

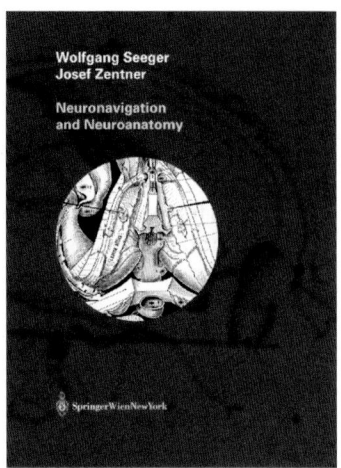

2002. VII, 419 pages. With 200 coloured figures.
Hardcover **EUR 248,–**
(Recommended retail price)
Net-price subject to local VAT.
ISBN 3-211-83741-8

Neuronavigation enables the surgeon to define each cranial and cerebral structure before and during surgery but the problem of brainshifting remains. This atlas shows drawings of anatomical landmarks for neuronavigation for preoperative planning. The authors show the relationships between bony landmarks which are unchanged during the operation, and landmarks which are no more available after opening of the skull but still recognizable during the operation, e.g. by ultrasonic sector scan. It further includes the description of many important anatomical variants, which are important for microsurgeons when using minimal invasive modern techniques (endoscopy, sterotaxy) to avoid errors and complications.

The book describes unknown projections for MRI and CT which may be adapted for special surgical problems. The anatomical drawings are the result of a twenty-five-years study of the topographical anatomy of the brain and the surrounding structures combined with the experience of modern microsurgery.

SpringerWienNewYork

P.O. Box 89, Sachsenplatz 4–6, 1201 Vienna, Austria, Fax +43.1.330 24 26, books@springer.at, **springer.at**
Haberstraße 7, 69126 Heidelberg, Germany, Fax +49.6221.345-4229, SDC-bookorder@springer.com, springer.com
P.O. Box 2485, Secaucus, NJ 07096-2485, USA, Fax +1.201.348-4505, service@springer-ny.com, springer.com
All errors and omissions excepted.

SpringerNeurosurgery

Wolfgang Seeger

Standard Variants of the Skull and Brain

Atlas for Neurosurgeons and
Neuroradiologists

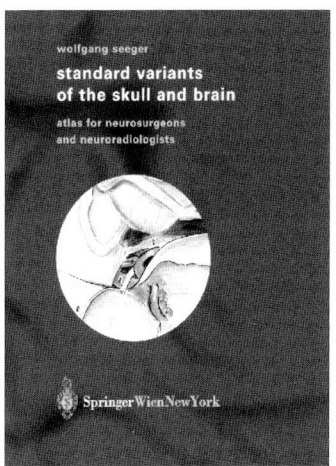

2003. VII, 371 pages. 177 figures, partly in colour.
Hardcover **EUR 230,–**
(Recommended retail price)
Net-price subject to local VAT.
ISBN 3-211-00956-6

The author describes in his unique style the anatomical variants of the brain and skull. This atlas is a continuation of his last work on „Neuronavigation and Neuroanatomy". Most anatomical reference volumes show a large number of common and rare variations. This atlas concentrates on well known and little known variants which are especially important for the clinicians, in particular the neurosurgeons and the radiologists. The variants have been grouped after areas of trepanation.

The author presents also a number of so far unknown variants gathered from his personal theoretical and clinical experience of 50 years. Exact knowledge of anatomical variations which the surgeon may encounter helps to plan operations and to avoid unexpected complications. Variants of no clinical relevance, even rather common ones, have not been included.

SpringerWien NewYork

P.O. Box 89, Sachsenplatz 4–6, 1201 Vienna, Austria, Fax +43.1.330 24 26, books@springer.at, **springer.at**
Haberstraße 7, 69126 Heidelberg, Germany, Fax +49.6221.345-4229, SDC-bookorder@springer.com, springer.com
P.O. Box 2485, Secaucus, NJ 07096-2485, USA, Fax +1.201.348-4505, service@springer-ny.com, springer.com
All errors and omissions excepted.

Springer and the Environment

WE AT SPRINGER FIRMLY BELIEVE THAT AN INTER-
national science publisher has a special obligation to
the environment, and our corporate policies consis-
tently reflect this conviction.

WE ALSO EXPECT OUR BUSINESS PARTNERS – PRINTERS,
paper mills, packaging manufacturers, etc. – to commit
themselves to using environmentally friendly materials and production processes.

THE PAPER IN THIS BOOK IS MADE FROM NO-CHLORINE
pulp and is acid free, in conformance with inter-
national standards for paper permanency.